Sam has a positive approach to treating people for stress, hypertension, headaches, weight control, and smoking.

Dr. Bernard Shostack, M.D.

Sam has had success with regard to weight control, stopping smoking, reducing stress and high blood pressure, and relieving headaches.

Dr. Donald M. Taylor, M.D.

Be What You Want to Be

HEAL YOURSELF

DARLENE NELSON

iUniverse, Inc.
Bloomington

Be What You Want to Be
Heal Yourself

Copyright © 2012 Darlene Nelson / Sam Meranto

iUniverse books may be ordered through booksellers or by contacting:

iUniverse
1663 Liberty Drive
Bloomington, IN 47403
www.iuniverse.com
1-800-Authors (1-800-288-4677)

ISBN: 978-1-4697-7822-8 (sc)
ISBN: 978-1-4697-7823-5 (hc)
ISBN: 978-1-4697-7824-2 (e)

Library of Congress Control Number: 2012903829

Printed in the United States of America

iUniverse rev. date: 7/3/2012

Contents

FOREWORD

Few books will change a person's life. The Bible is one, and this new book of Sam's is another. I have been in ministry for four decades, in education all my life, and in psychology and sociology for three decades. I can tell you, Sam's esoteric methods work brilliantly! I have learned more in sessions from Sam than I have from hundreds if not thousands of books or lectures, because they access a side of the brain rarely used or even explored. This is what makes Sam a pioneer in his field. Under Sam's sessions this summer, I can state my mind is allowing greater efficiency in maintaining a 98 percent overall and 3.97 GPA in the doctoral community program I attend. I have also lost weight and medaled four times in marathons this summer. That is a good feat for a man in his mid-fifties.

Truly, Sam is a man well ahead of his time and a well-kept secret. No matter what walk of life, what faith you may be, or what issue you may have, you can find comfort, solace, and the help you need within the first words and techniques of this book.

May the Lord bless you and your family and the friends with whom you share this book. If you are in the Phoenix, Arizona, area, come on in and meet Sam personally. You may have discovered the magic of the eighth wonder of the world right here. He is so excited to meet new people, he offers them a $300 session free just for coming by.

Dr. Joseph Gering

Sam Meranto

Who is Sam Meranto? Sam has been called "the fastest, most successful therapist that ever lived by his clients." In 1978 Sam was granted a doctorate in the field of medical hypnosis (DH) by Maryland State Homeopathic Medical Society. In my personal opinion, Sam is truly a gift from God.

God saved Sam Meranto's life from a tornado on June 9, 1953, in Worcester, Massachusetts. Ninety people died where he was standing, and over ten thousand were injured. It was the tenth worst tornado in US history. I believe God saved Sam's life so he could do the work he is doing today.

When I share stories of people Sam has helped, many I have had the opportunity to hear firsthand, you can understand why I am so passionate to share Sam's extraordinary abilities and what he can do for you.

At the end of this book, I will share a handful of pictures and stories about clients Sam helped: people who had lost all hope until they enrolled in Sam's program. Some of these people had seen up to thirty doctors, been in as many as four famous hospitals, and even been to faith healers with no help. Sam was their last hope. In a matter of six minutes (yes, six minutes), Sam was able to get to the root of their problem and begin the process to help them. Their stories are so incredible I have put them in a link for you to log onto and hear for yourself at http://www.youtube.com/smeranto.

Sam's ability to find the root of a person's problem is truly a gift from God. These solutions to people's problems seem to come to Sam automatically from above. The problems are usually so simple that nobody can find them. It's like the nose on your face: you can't see it unless you look in a mirror. After Sam finds the problem, he guides the client into curing himself or herself. That's what I call a miracle from God.

According to the Bible, it took God six days to make the world, and He rested on the seventh. If God can create the whole world in only six days, why should it take years and years for people to get help with psychological problems? I read that the average psychiatrist treats only four to five hundred patients in a thirty-year career. This means he or she only sees an average of thirteen to seventeen patients a year! That's because each patient sees the doctor once or twice a week for years and years, talking about the same problems on every visit. Most of them get worse instead of better. They keep going to the doctor year after year to get their prescriptions, because now they are dependent on them. In fact, the Arizona Republic did a story by United Press International (January 4, 1985) titled "ex-psychiatric patients' death rate is surprisingly high, researchers find".

Sam had a psychiatrist, Dr. Norys, come to him. He said in the last thirty years, he had treated all sorts of people, mostly by prescribing medication. Dr. Norys went through a divorce and was upset and depressed, so he decided to enroll in Sam's program. He asked Sam what he thought of psychiatrists. Sam said, "They are all good, and they mean well." That's when Dr. Norys admitted to Sam that he was a psychiatrist and wasn't happy with the training he received. He was amazed at the results Sam's clients were receiving.

Sam introduced the doctor to many of his clients, and Dr. Norys was bewildered and amazed. He asked, "You do all this without medication?"

And Sam's response was, "The Bible has all the answers. It states, 'A [happy] cheerful heart is good medicine,' in Proverbs 17:22 (NIB). Give people a solution to their problems, and God will do the rest."

Dr. Norys then told Sam, "You should start a school to train doctors guided meditation. Their medical training is not getting the job done."

In just two weeks, Dr. Norys felt like a new man. Sam videotaped him making this statement, which I have personally heard. Dr. Norys said, "I've learned more in two weeks on your program than all my medical training and thirty years in practice."

Sam wants to make it very clear that what he does he does not call a practice. Ballplayers practice and then they play ball. We're playing ball and getting the job done with God's help and guidance. Sam doesn't just look at a base hit; he looks at the home run—the whole picture of fixing the root of the problem. If you just put a Band-Aid on a problem, the problem will keep coming back. This is why Sam's program is so successful. He gets to the root of the issues and removes it for permanent results.

The following story was written by John Pritchard, a researcher who wanted to discredit what Sam did. I found it so powerful that I wanted to share it with you.

One of the world's greatest inventors, Thomas Alva Edison, in his declining years, told reporters on several occasions before his death, according to the *World Book Encyclopedia,* "I am working on a device so sensitive that if there is life after death it will pick up the evidence of it."

The same data source says that out of his more than one thousand inventions no one, before now, has been able to find out if the device he spoke of exists. I believe I have accidentally discovered the invention Edison talked about.

I've been watching a Phoenix, Arizona, spiritual meditation expert and scores of his subjects on his weekly TV shows. As I have watched and listened to testimonials of Sam Meranto's clients, their stories are unbelievable! I believe that Sam has been using the device that Thomas Edison invented. In the office, too, is a large photo taken over fifty years ago of Meranto holding up an electric lightbulb, Edison's most famous invention, as the focal object to mesmerize a girl.

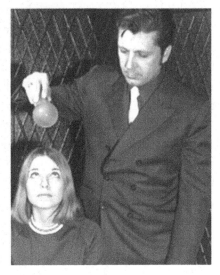

Why a lightbulb? He could have chosen a ring, a pen, a coin, or a twirling watch. That photo aroused my curiosity. I learned that Meranto was born in 1931, a date I recalled as having some historical significance, but I couldn't think what it was at that moment.

As I've watched and listened to the testimonials of Sam Meranto's clients, their stories are unbelievable. People with cancer, leukemia, and mysterious diseases: some have been treated by as many as thirty medical doctors, faith healers, and have been in and out of all kinds of hospitals, such as UCLA Medical Center, Scripps Diagnostic Clinic, Ann Arbor Hospital, Mayo Clinic, and many others. They were told, "There is nothing more medical science can do for you." They came to Sam Meranto as a last resort, and they got help by listening to Sam's spiritual meditation sessions on audio recordings. Now, how can this man get those results by just listening to his voice? So, I started investigating to see if he was for real or a fake.

After hearing those testimonials of miraculous help from the spiritual meditation expert, I made an appointment and went to Sam Meranto's office with the intent of exposing him as a fraud. There, thinking of me as a potential client, he introduced me to many members of his Think Faith Center. Each one of them told me about dramatic help that Sam has given them. One man had lost 225 excess pounds.

I met senior citizens who have given up crutches and walkers. I saw children who were born with physical problems and who are now attending regular schools. And I met former heroin and crystal meth addicts who said Sam had helped them get those monkeys off their backs after being in $8,000 rehabilitation programs that had failed. But even after talking with all of those people face to face, I remained a skeptic in search of a story to expose the fakery of Sam Meranto.

I told him I was interested in his program but avoided signing up right away. I returned to his center several times, met more of his clients, and heard more tales of miraculous help. Finally, I told Sam right out: I was there to write a story about him as a fraud. He surprised me by not being upset. He said, "I don't blame you for thinking that way. It's hard to believe that my helping these people could accomplish so many miracles."

I asked him if he would cooperate with me by answering questions about his background, his use of meditation, and his work today. He agreed without hesitation.

Sam Meranto took time to show me through his center. I saw his state-of-the-art television studio. In his office, there is almost every device that Thomas Edison invented.

I also learned that in 1953, in Worcester, Massachusetts, Sam was standing where a tornado struck, killing ninety people and injuring thousands. Sam walked away not more than three minutes before it struck. Sam feels God saved him to do the work he is doing today.

He showed me his antique wire voice recorder, Edison's favorite invention, that he bought years ago to make recordings to help salespeople boost their productivity.

Delving further into Meranto's life, he told me he'd learned about meditation in Massachusetts while still a teenager. In 1956, he started teaching medical doctors how to use meditation to help their patients with weight loss, to stop smoking, to treat stress, depression, and sex and skin problems. He showed me the, "Thanks for teaching me," letters from doctors he had taught.

That evening I reviewed the notes I'd made at Meranto's Center and thought about the things he'd shown me that he uses in his work, every one a Thomas Edison invention.

Thinking again about the photo in his office—Meranto as a young man, using an Edison-invented lightbulb as his meditation focal object—I wonder if perhaps I'm onto something unusual?

Looking up "Edison" in my encyclopedia, I began to read about his life and inventions. I can hardly believe what I'm reading, and the photo there—of young Edison beside his wax voice recorder—why, he looks exactly like young Meranto, holding up the lightbulb. Reading on, I recognize that things Thomas Edison and Sam Meranto share in common are far too many to be pure coincidence. It's mind-boggling.

Sam wants to make this perfectly clear. He does not think he is Edison. He calls it just a coincidence. As a reporter, I believe differently. If there is a past life, this definitely is Edison here to help humanity.

Could Edison be here, helping us with our problems? Sam says, "The only thing he is helping me with is by inventing the tools I use."

Sam Meranto does not like the word "hypnosis." Most people think you are going to make them act like a chicken or a dog.

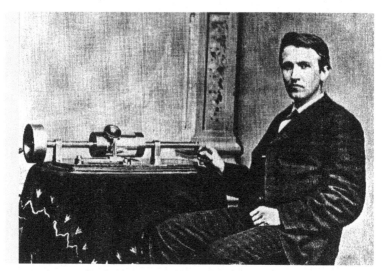

Picture of Edison - courtesy of National Park Services

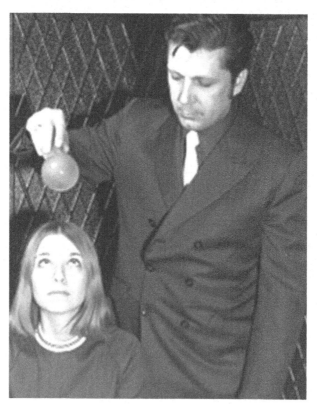

Edison looks like young Meranto holding up the light bulb.

The Bible makes it clear not to believe in fortune-tellers or people that take control over our mind. The Bible does state, "Lay down in your bed close your eyes, meditate, and open your mind to the Lord" (Psalms 4:8, 63:6). Sam is an ordained minister, and he is working for the Lord. Actually, he is dehypnotizing God's children from pain, depression, gluttony, smoking, drinking, reliance on prescription or illegal drugs, getting over the loss of a loved one, divorces, and physical and sexual abuse. This truly is the Lord's work. Sam gives God the credit for all of the miracles that he has helped perform in the name of God, the Holy Spirit, and in the name of Jesus for Christians.

Edison died on October 18, 1931, in New Jersey of a respiratory ailment. Sam Meranto was born sixteen days later, on November 3, 1931, a few miles away, in New York State with an infant's respiratory ailment.

Edison's father and his grandfather were both named Sam. Was it foreordained or coincidence that Meranto was named Sam at birth? Edison's mother was born in Canada. Sam's mother was born in Canada; another coincidence?

Earlier that day, Sam had told me that he'd always wanted to be an inventor. He showed me his two US patents issued for his inventions. His first patent was issued in 1967. Edison finished his first invention to become patented in 1867, *exactly one hundred years before.*

Meranto holds his second patent, but he was not destined to be a great inventor. That, in itself, poses a significant question. If an outstanding inventor comes back into our world, does he return with the same talents of his previous life, or does he come back with "spin-off" talents, such as being able to demonstrate masterful use of things he invented in his previous life?

Sam Meranto is no prolific inventor, but it is evident, by results he gets for clients, that he is loaded with *extraordinary abilities* to utilize Edison inventions. Hospitals, therapists, psychiatrists, and psychologists each use voice recorders in their practices, but none of them, as far as I have been able to determine, get the consistent positive results that Sam Meranto gets with the voice recorder, Edison's favorite invention.

There are many more similarities shared by Edison and Meranto. Edison spent three months in school, and the teacher sent him home, telling his mother that he was incapable of learning; that he asked too many questions. Meranto was sent home from school repeatedly because he talked too much and asked too many questions. Coincidence? Let's go further.

Meranto was dehypnotizing people in the Arizona sunshine in 1978, attempting to harness the sun's energy for weight reduction. Phoenix TV station Channel 10 made a news feature of his effort, and the *Phoenix Gazette* published a feature article about what he was doing, headed, "Valley Sun 'Burns off Weight'."

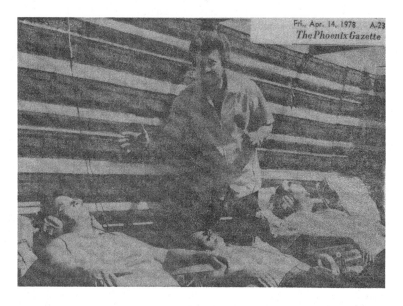

Precisely one hundred years before, in 1878, Thomas Edison was working on a project to harness the sun's energy. Coincidence? Perhaps.

Then let's add these facts, too. Edison was married twice and had six children. Meranto has been married twice and had six children.

One of my questions to Meranto was, "What sports do you like?" His reply was that he has no time for sports and spends most of his time trying to help people solve problems. He added, however, that he does sometimes shoot pool on his table at home. While reading about Edison, I discovered that he disliked sports, thinking them a waste of time, but that he did enjoy using the pool table in his home. Another coincidence.

Meranto's weakness is that he craves a good cigar every once in a while. Edison, according to the encyclopedia, was a frequent cigar smoker.

Both men show the Edison patience in their work (but not always so in the personal aspects of their lives). Edison is reported to have experienced over ten thousand failures while trying to make a working battery for automobiles. When told if he kept better records he could have saved years of time and thousands of experiments in developing that product, he replied, "I have not failed. I've just found 10,000 ways that won't work." By Satender 24 Jul 2011at simple4job.com.

Meranto's work patience has allowed him to produce more than seventeen hundred different audio recordings to help people with almost any problem, real or imagined. He told me that he made every one of them without a script or an outline. He simply picks up his microphone, another Edison invention, and makes an audio recording nonstop, while what needs to be on it comes into his mind.

Both Thomas A. Edison, inventor, and Sam Meranto, spiritual meditation expert and master user of Edison's inventions, were essentially self-educated. They learned through reading, experimentation, and doing. There are so many similarities shared by the two men that it's awesome. Is Sam Meranto, indeed, Thomas Edison back among us, proving there is life after death?

Meranto has voice recorders or video cameras in every room of his center. Sam even has an audio record of the very first time Edison allowed himself to be recorded over eighty years ago.

The day after my evening of discovering these tremendous numbers of similarities shared by Edison and Meranto, I returned to Sam's Center to ask him, "Do you think you might be the reincarnation of Edison back on earth or that his spirit is guiding you?"

Meranto smiled and then replied, "God gave me the gift and the talent to help people. I don't believe in reincarnation or spirits coming back to guide somebody."

Sam said, "I have to admit when I look at some of the similarities, chills run up and down my back. I remember when I was five years old. I got behind a stand-up radio and started pulling all the tubes out. They were all over the floor. My father and mother had a fit.

"I have always been fascinated with cameras and radios. I went to a theater when I was five years old with my sister, Margaret, to see a western starring Tom Mix and Buck Jones. I had my first little camera and I was trying to take pictures of the movie screen. When I was twenty, I won a Brownie 8mm movie camera as top salesman. I have closets full of movies I took of my kids. I guess I just like gadgets. People would ask me if I believed in past lives, and if so, who did I think I was. Jokingly, I would say Thomas Edison. But I was only kidding at the time, I didn't know about the similarities. If you ask me, it is scary. But I don't want people to think I am a weirdo, believing in such nonsense. I do feel there is a higher spirit coming from God that's been guiding me into helping people in need."

In my opinion as a research author, I started off to prove Sam Meranto as a fake. Much to my amazement,

I found Sam Meranto to be a genuine genius.

How do you account for his success with the public? Sam is able to find the problem after some patients have been to as many as thirty doctors, and they did not get the help they wanted. Some of these patients were told that medical science has done all they can. Here is a letter from Dr. Shostack, MD, from 1978. He states that a man with colitis that has tried everything to no avail got positive results with Sam Meranto.

BERNARD SHOSTACK, M.D.
3417 NORTH 32ND STREET
PHOENIX, ARIZONA 85018

GENERAL FAMILY PRACTICE

DAY OR NIGHT
(602) 956-7740

August 6, 1982

Re: Sam Meranto

To Whom It May Concern:

Mr. Meranto is known to me since 1978, when he opened an office for weight control and smoking on Indian School Road.

Since that time, we have observed the results of his behaviour modification techniques on a number of patients. He has had a positive approach to treating people for stress, hypertension, headaches, weight control and smoking. He has done this by direct treatment and by the use of cassette tapes. In one particular patient of mine, he was extremely successful in treatment of colitis. This had been after a number of failures by other modalities of treatment.

He is of good character and honest in his approach to treatment of his clients and I would have no hesitation in referring the appropriate problems to him.

Sincerely,

B. Shostack, M.D.

BS/js

13

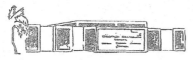

MOUNTAIN VIEW MEDICAL CLINIC LTD.   4600 E. Indian School Rd. • Phoenix, Arizona 85018 • Phone 959-175t

FAMILY PHYSICIANS
GENNARO LICOSATI, M.D.   CHARLES L. LEVISON, M.D.   JOHN W. CURTIN, M.D.   DONALD M. TAYLOR, M.D.   MICHAEL J. LIPSON, M.D.

July 23, 1982

RE: Sam Meranto

TO WHOM IT MAY CONCERN:

This letter is to state that I have known Mr. Sam Meranto since 1978 and we have worked together during that time. I have referred my patients to him and have seen people who have been to his center.

In that four year time period, I have observed very positive results from Sam's sessions with the behavior modification think tapes. He has had success with regard to weight control, stopping smoking, reducing stress and high blood pressure and relieving headaches.

If I may provide any further documentation of Sam Meranto's good character and professional attitude, please contact me and I will be happy to comply.

Sincerely,

Donald M. Taylor, M.D.

DMT:smk

14

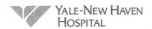

June 7, 2007

Sam Meranto
4440 East Indian School Road
Phoenix, AZ 85018

Dear Mr. Meranto:

On behalf of the Elder Horizons Program at Yale New Haven
Hospital, I would like to thank you for your generous gift of tapes and
CD's covering weight loss, depression, pain, stress and healing. I am
sure the tapes and CDs will be of great use.

Again, thank you for the generous contribution to our program.

Sincerely,

Susann Varano, MD
Director, Elder Horizons Program
Yale New Haven Hospital

20 York Street
New Haven, CT 06510-3202

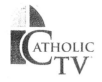

May 29, 2009

Dear Sam:

I would like to take the time to thank you. When I first met you nine years ago at PAX TV's convention, it must have been God that put you and your lovely wife at my dinner table.

I told you I had a brain tumor. The doctors said I had to go in for an operation. The tumor was growing larger every month. You reached over, put your hands on my head and said a prayer. You asked God to stop the tumor from growing in the name of Jesus.
I went back to the doctors and the tumor quit growing. It has been nine years now, Praise the Lord. I have to mention that I have been prayed for many times with no results. You must have a direct connection with the Lord. May God bless you and your ministry.

I will be in Phoenix August 2nd, putting on a seminar for the Knights of Columbus. You have my cell number: 1-617-448-7086. I would love to see you and your wife again when I am in Phoenix.

Sincerely,

Steve Sasso

The Salvation Army

FOUNDED 1865
2707 EAST VAN BUREN STREET
P.O. BOX 13107   •   PHONE (602) 267-4100
PHOENIX, ARIZONA 85002

Memorandum

November 1, 1989

Dear Mr. Meranto:

Thank you for taking the time to speak yesterday to Burdell and myself. He has much admiration for you and the work you have done. His state of being shows the accomplishments that can be done with mind power.

As per our conversation, you stated you would be willing to donate tapes to the Salvation Army Motivated Adult Program for our use with the people who need our help. I would most certainly like to thank you for this gesture as your work has been admired by myself and countless people since you began your career in the healing of the mind power.

Mr. Groen has had praises for your part in his recovery and the state of his health as it is today. He has certainly had a turn around in his life, and much of the thanks go to you because o his use of your tapes.

God Bless you Sam, and most certainly keep up the good deeds.

Alice M. Kirby
Counsler, Salvation Army

17

Hospitals, therapists, psychiatrists, and psychologists each use voice recorders in their practices, but none of them, as far as I have been able to determine, get the consistent positive results that Sam Meranto gets!

John Pritchard

It Begins in the Womb

Decades before others started to talk about how the first nine months in the womb shape the rest of your life, Sam was already using this information as a vital factor in his program. TIME magazine had a featured cover on this (October 4, 2010).

The most important part of your life is your childhood. It starts right in your mother's womb, while she is carrying you. You have heard of crack babies and alcoholic babies. These babies tasted these chemicals and alcohol through the umbilical cord. At forty-five days of conception, the brain is developed. In three months, the complete body is formed. The baby experiences everything the mother is going through; that's why some adopted children have a lot of psychological problems, and children that come from parents that argued a lot. Sam's program can benefit them substantially. Sam shared true stories with me of actual patients he helped who had depression all their lives because of something that happened while they were being formed in the womb.

One of his clients, Malachai, a thirty-eight-year-old schoolteacher and ex-pro football player, had depression since his childhood. He saw as many as fifteen doctors, tried all kinds of prescriptions, including the so-called happy pills, which we know have been known to cause violence and suicide in some people. He came into Sam's office to tell him how great he felt for the first time in years! He was even on one of Sam's television infomercials. He came mainly to give encouragement to other people who are suffering. He had seen a previous infomercial that encouraged him to get some help. He wanted to do the same for someone else.

Sam asked him if his mother had any problems while carrying him in the womb. He said, "None that I know of." Sam asked if his mother was still alive. He said, "Yes, she lives in Chicago." Then, Sam asked him to pick up his office phone and call her right then. Malachai dialed his mother's number. When she answered, he asked, "Mom, did you have any problems while carrying me, when you were pregnant?" There was a silence. He kept asking, "Ma, Ma, are you there?"

Finally, she answered, "Why do you ask?"

He said, "I'm with Sam Meranto, and he is helping me with depression. You know that I've had depression for years."

Malachai's mother said, "I didn't want to tell you this. I didn't want to be pregnant again. And I cried every day when I was pregnant with you. However, after you were born, I was glad and very happy. I love you very much, and I'm so proud of you." The problem was deep-seated. After he listened to sessions Sam made for this kind of problem, Malachai is now a much happier person.

Sam had clients who, while in a relaxed state, recalled their mother trying to abort them with a coat hanger!

One morning in the eighties, Sam recalled watching *Good Morning America*, hosted by David Hartman. David was interviewing a woman who had a sixteen-year-old son who played three musical instruments, graduated from college and medical school, and was a medical doctor, going through his internship. Can you imagine a sixteen-year-old as a medical doctor? Now this got Sam's curiosity, so he stayed up to watch the entire broadcast. David Hartman asked her, "You have two other children who are average. What did you do different to get a genius?"

She replied, "With the first two children, I had to work. With the last child, we were financially secure. I didn't have to work. I stayed home and played the piano. I would read all kinds of books. I would rest the book on my stomach while I read. I'd feel him kicking the book, and I would talk to him as if he was there. I would tell him how smart he was going to be. I'd even put music on and danced around the house with a broom. My husband would come home and put his hand on my stomach and talk to him. That was all I did that was different with my last child. It's funny: my other two children have very good business sense. Could they have picked that up while I was working and running a business?"

If you are expecting a child or have a friend or a relative who is expecting, talk to your child while they are in the womb, read books to them, and tell your friends who are expecting a child to do the same.

Sam has four grandchildren. He instructed his daughter-in law, while she was carrying her children, to do the same. His grandson Anthony is ten years old. He plays the violin, speaks some Spanish, and is an A+ student. His granddaughter, Alexi, just got a beautiful report card showing she is the top student in her class. Her teachers say she is a delight to have as a pupil, and she is only eight years old. Joey just turned six and got almost the same response from his teacher. The oldest grandson, Franky, is now thirteen. He is from Sam's son's first marriage. Franky was a slow learner and had a behavior problem. His birth mother didn't have the benefit of Grandpa's wisdom. However, Franky is doing much better now. Sam gave him some of his sessions, and his marks in school have skyrocketed. His teacher can't believe the difference in his schoolwork and especially in his behavior.

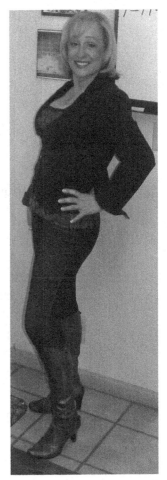

I encourage anyone having a problem with a child to check out Sam's program. Sam has prerecorded sessions that can be mailed to them. Sam even has sessions for bed-wetting, being overweight (which is horribly on the rise), in addition to smoking, drug addiction, and bullying. You name it, and Sam has done a program for it! I am excited to brag, being a personal recipient of the benefits of Sam's program. Sam has personally helped me with weight loss, depression, and a multitude of other issues.

The first nine months in the womb shape the rest of your life!

Sam Meranto

READ AND TRANCE AWAY YOUR PROBLEMS

Hello. I'm Tony Evans. I've known Sam Meranto for over twenty years. I've personally seen miracles that people have received by listening to his famous audios and watching his videos. Sam is the only one I know who does all of his recordings without a script. He has recorded over seventeen hundred sessions, covering all subjects. What makes Sam special is he simplifies things and does not make them complicated. He holds three US patents, and with his inventive mind and remarkable gifts, he has pioneered a new approach that releases people from problems and difficulties they have struggled with for years. Many of his clients have been to universities, hospitals, faith healers, and all kinds of doctors without getting the help they wanted. Even psychiatrists, psychologists, and professors have come to him for personal help. Sam sessions go far beyond educating you. They deal with your problems in a very powerful way.

Sam was born in Niagara Falls, New York, in 1931. He started studying the mind in 1952, with Doctor Rexford L. North in Boston, Massachusetts. That gives him over fifty years of experience.

Yale Hospital in Connecticut has used his sessions in their senior care program and was well received. Tucson Medical Center has used his sessions for severe pain.

And now, I give you the creator of the Power Within—Sam Meranto.

Thank you, Tony. I took a class in New York City with a Doctor Bryan. F. Lee Bailey, a brilliant trial attorney, was there. We had a class on the power of the mind. We took people who were deaf and put them in a trance by holding scorecards. We would hold up a card that said, "Keep your eyes open and relax." Another card would say, "Your arms are getting heavy. Keep your eyes open. Your legs are getting heavy." People were put in a trance with their eyes open. They got results for weight loss, depression, pain, alcoholism, drug addiction, and motivation. These were people who could not hear—some not even a sound.

So today, I am going to make a session that you can read and get benefits from, just like if you were put in a trance. Have you heard of road hypnosis (white line fever)? As a person drives down the road, staring at the white line in the center of the road, he or she can go into a trance. These individuals can end up in serious accidents. We want you to read this book. Keep your eyes wide open. Sit in a nice, comfortable place or lie on a couch or bed. You could be reading this in a hospital. I am going to put you into a trance state, and your eyes will stay open.

I made a session for tractor-trailer drivers who drink a lot of coffee, because they are trying to stay awake for hours. Some drive for eleven hours at a time. So, I made a session telling them that while their hands were on the steering wheel, their eyes were locked open, and they would be safe, courteous drivers. It worked like a charm. They didn't need to have that coffee poured into them like they had been doing to try to stay awake.

I want you to stay wide-awake. Get relaxed while reading this book, and you will experience some beautiful things. You are going to feel happier. You're not going worry as much as you have been. Worry never solved the problem. It only makes it worse. So, while your hands are on the book, your eyes are wide open. You are alert subconsciously. You see, you have one brain and two compartments: the conscious compartment and the subconscious compartment. You consciously picked up this book and started to read it. Suggestions are going to put your conscious mind to sleep. Subconsciously, you're going to be wide-awake. Therefore, we can make some changes in the back of your mind. You can get benefits from reading this book.

This will be the first book that can actually give you therapy while reading it. Most books people buy that talk about psychology and psychiatry talk about what you should do and what you shouldn't do. These books have proven to get very little results.

You keep your eyes on the pages and your eyes will be locked open while you are reading. Consciously, you're going to fall asleep. In their sleep, mothers can hear a baby crying and wake up automatically. They program themselves for that. When you read these pages, your arms will start to get very relaxed. You're going to feel very sleepy. Your conscious mind will fall asleep. Subconsciously, you will be wide-awake and alert. Mothers wake up from a sound sleep because subconsciously, they are awake twenty-four hours a day. You don't roll out of bed at night. Why is that? When you were a baby, your mother put you in a crib with railings and padding, and you bumped your head when you rolled over. Each time you bumped your head, it programmed your subconscious mind not to roll out of your bed. After about two years, mothers take the railings away, and you never roll out of bed. It took you two years to be programmed.

A lot of people have been programmed three times a day for an average of eighteen years: clean your plate, don't waste your food, kids are starving in other countries; I'll tell your father if you don't eat all your food. It becomes deeply embedded in the back of your subconscious. You can become a dietician, a doctor, or anything you want to become, yet you'll still eat the way you've been programmed. You've had eighteen years of programming by people who loved you, cared about you, and wanted you to grow big and strong. They didn't know about nutrition like they know today. In the back of our subconscious mind we eat too much food. We clean the plate even though we are full. According to U.S. News & World Reports "The one antiaging remedy that works: reducing food intake by 40 percent" (August 18-25, 1997 page 57 by Nancy Shute). In The Arizona Republic newspaper Nanci Hellmich wrote 100,500 cancer cases a year linked to obesity (11/05/2009).

Your conscious mind can be your own worst enemy. Consciously people tell themselves they can't do this or that. "I'll never get ahead." "I don't get the breaks." They have been programmed to think that way. A lot has to do with their childhood and who raised them.

I have sessions that can actually improve your life 100 percent. Your mind is a computer. It is God's computer. When you are reading this, your body feels relaxed. You feel tranquil and start to take deep breaths. I want these written words to flow into your subconscious mind. You will find yourself making some lifestyle changes. Can you imagine how powerful it would be to listen to my sessions? It is so powerful. It is almost like you went and bought a new brain.

My sessions take advantage of your senses. When you smell something like lilacs, you can tell. When you smell gasoline, you can tell what that is. You smell nice odors and bad odors. The smell goes to the brain, and you know what it is. Somebody hugs you, and you feel his or her love. Somebody hits you, and you feel the person's anger. Your brain interprets what's going on. You see beautiful things. You see some disasters, especially on television. You see some terrible things. Your brain interprets them. You taste food and know if it is a lemon or an onion. Your sub-conscious tells you the difference because when you started off eating as a youngster the tastes were recorded. Your mind is a computer. It gives you a playback. I make sessions that you can hear, so if you have a vision problem, you can still get the benefits by listening versus reading.

As I said before, this is the first written book that's actually going to put you into a trance. I don't want to call it hypnosis. The word "hypnosis" is a Greek word. It means to sleep artificially induced. I hate that word. People think you are going to make them act like a chicken or a dog. They think you are going to take control of their minds. I call it meditation. It is written in the Bible in Psalms 4:4 to lie down in your bed, close your eyes and meditate and open your mind to the Lord. The Lord wants me to write this book, so you can meditate with your eyes open.

Looking into a fireplace can put you into a relaxed trance state. A flicker of a candle can put you into a relaxed trance state. Looking out at the ocean, with the waves splashing against the shore, can put you into a relaxed state. Now, reading this book can put you into a relaxed state. When you flip the pages, you will go deeper and deeper into a relaxed state.

You know who the world's greatest hypnotist is. Well, if you really want to get technical, God created Adam and Eve. He put Adam into a deep, deep sleep and took a rib and made Eve. So, he is probably the first one who put a person into a deep sleep.

Mothers are great hypnotists. Example: they sing "Rock a bye baby, on the treetop. When the wind blows, the cradle will rock." Mothers have had hypnotic powers over their children since the beginning of time. They have hypnotic power over us. After all, we came from within her. A lot of mothers gave beautiful programming to their children. But God forbid your mother had a bad childhood. If a mother was abused when she was young, she could program her children in a negative way without realizing it. "You're just like your father." "You'll never amount to anything." "What's wrong with you? Are you stupid?" I'm not saying all mothers have done this, but some mothers that have been mistreated in their childhood with depression have. The Bible states, "Honor your Father and mother." (Ephesians 6:2 KJV). That doesn't mean you have to like some of the things they did to you. If you had a problem with your father or mother, check on their childhood, and you will often find out he or she had worse problems than you while they were growing up. Therefore, it is second nature to them to program their children in a negative way.

The sessions I make have no written script. I just sit by the microphones and call on the good Lord above to guide me into what he wants people to hear. I've made almost sixteen hundred sessions to date. We have people fill out a questionnaire and evaluation of 225 questions, which they send to our headquarters in Phoenix, Arizona. We analyze it. Keep your eyes open while you're reading this book. Feel your legs, your arms, and feel yourself just relaxing. You feel so drowsy, so sleepy. And now, to get back to the evaluation they fill out and send to us. We will know more about the person than he or she knows about himself or herself. The form is available as a free download at sammeranto.com.

I had a client who was a professor from ASU, where he had taught psychology for thirty years. His name is Doctor Beard. He came into my office and said, "I've been hearing about you from my students. I drive by your office most every day going to ASU in Tempe. I have depression. I have been taking medication for years and been to many of my colleagues. And I don't know what is wrong with me." He wrote an article about me. In fact, it is in back of the evaluation you can download for free.

His story can help you. His mother was a professor. She was tough on him and always found fault with him. She'd grab him when was small—about five years old or so—and tell him, "You are going to be a professor like me." His father left and divorced his mother. So, he was stuck with his mother, who was angry because her husband had left her.

He admitted to me his grandmother was something like her. See, how we react is passed from one generation to the next.

When he came to me, I said, "I found your problem, and it took me less than six minutes. Your mother was tough on you and found fault with you. Your father was smart; he got out of the house. But you were stuck there." His mother never celebrated Christmas, because how can you be happy when your husband leaves you? When he got through my program, he came into my office dressed as Santa Claus, smiling; we shot some pictures with him. He said, "I've never laughed. I never smiled before. I've always taken things too seriously. I was never getting things done, because my mother told me I never finish anything."

I said, "You became a professor. You had to finish school."

He said, "That was a job. I start projects, and I don't finish them." He came to me after he had his been in the program for a while. He said, "I finish things; I get it done now. It's so beautiful. Everything has changed."

Folks, I am a self-educated man. I've had some training from William Brian, M.D. from the American Medical College of Hypnosis. That's where I took classes, and F. Lee Bailey, one of the most famous trial attorneys in the country at that time was there. What I do is a gift: a gift from God. Elvis Presley never had a lesson. Einstein: look at what he accomplished as a self-educated individual. Thomas Edison, too. I used to joke if there was a past life, I was probably Thomas Edison. I was just joking, until a guy wrote a story about it. It kind of amazed me. I denied the whole story, of course. I don't want people thinking I'm a weirdo. But I'm using his lights right now. I'm using his microphones right now. He perfected the first motion picture camera, and now we have a video camera. It's strange.

You who are reading this have a gift, too. You have a natural talent and a natural ability that you have not been using the way you should. You will start to develop your natural talents and abilities. Stop telling yourself you can't. Stop telling yourself you don't have enough education. You didn't finish school. Did you know some of the wealthiest men who ever lived were self-educated? Thomas Edison spent three months in school, and they sent him home. They said he was incapable of learning. His mother had to teach him.

Henry Ford, one of Edison's friends, went to the fifth grade. He went to court one time, and the lawyer was asking him all kinds of questions. Henry kept saying, "I don't know."

The lawyer said, "What do you mean, you don't know? You run this big company."

Henry said, "I hire guys like you for a dime a dozen to do that stuff for me." (Think and grow rich by Napoleon Hill).

Henry Ford had a vision. Do you have a vision? Do you look into the future and see yourself successful, whether it's at weight loss or stopping alcohol or drug abuse? I'm giving you written suggestions that are just as powerful as the spoken word: you are special and unique. You can make things happen. I don't want to hear the excuse you came from a poor family or you don't have enough education. There are so many men and women who have accomplished unbelievable things with a natural gift they received from our maker, and that's the good Lord above. You have been hypnotized into failing. I call myself a dehypnotist, because you've convinced yourself—and others have convinced you—that you have a problem. I help you undo that hypnosis.

I want to mention this to you: there is a lot of problems with drugs and alcohol. Get relaxed while you are reading this book. Feel your arms and legs relaxing. Feel your conscious mind going to sleep. We are right in the back of your gold mine, right in the back of your subconscious mind, pulling out your natural talents and your natural abilities. Learn how to tap the powers you have.

I had a lady come into my office. She said she spent $40,000 she borrowed from her brother to go to the Meadows in Wickenburg, Arizona. They specialized in alcohol and drug addictions. She said, "I spent thirty-six days there. I had the best of foods. I met a lot of nice people there. I was out three weeks, and I got together with some other people I met there. These are rich people who can afford $40,000 for a thirty-six-day treatment. We all got drunk out of our minds." Three weeks after she left the Meadows, she enrolled in my program, and I gave her some CDs to take with her. She signed to do a regression, where I work with her personally. I called her up a few months later and said, "Come on into the office. I am going to work with you personally."

She said, "You don't have to. All my friends cannot believe me. I can sit there and watch them drink. I don't want to drink anymore." How in the world can someone spend $40,000 for thirty-six days and come to me and—for practically nothing—stop drinking alcohol. The reason for that is I get into the back of your brain, where your problem is deep-seated.

I had another guy, who was from Austria. He said, "You stopped my wife from smoking cigarettes." And she's been to hypnotists. She's been to Asia. She's been to psychiatrists. She's been trying to stop for years and years. He said, "She doesn't smoke anymore. She owns a bar, where they all sit in the back and smoke, and she goes out there, joins them, and watches them smoke. She used to smoke two packs a day." That's over $5,800 in cigarettes a year at two packs a day for $8 a pack. He asked, "Do you think you can help me? I'm in charge of the Navajo Indian casinos setting up their bars and restaurants. They love me there. I've already spent over $200,000. I've been in three hospitals and seven clinics all together. I can't stop drinking. But you stopped my wife from smoking, so maybe you can help me." He enrolled in my program to do a regression. I called him up. He said, "Sam, I went back to Austria, and they threw a party for me. Everybody had drinks and Vodka and everything. I sat down with a little soda water and lime. I didn't have a drink, and I loved it." The guy spent over $200,000 to stop alcoholism.

I want you, as you read this, to feel a tingling in the palms of your hands. And feel a tingling in your fingers, especially when you turn the pages of this book. Feel yourself just relaxing. Consciously, you are falling into a sleep like state. But you will be wide-awake subconsciously. People dream, talk in their sleep, and sleepwalk. I've had people tell me they find dirty dishes, but there is nobody in the house but them. They don't even remember getting up and eating. There are cigarette butts in the ashtrays, and they don't remember getting up and smoking. Your subconscious is alive. You tap the power of your subconscious mind, and you can do anything you want to do. You can even improve your health when you read this book. I want you to get something out of reading this portion of the book. I want you to smile more. I want you to feel happier. I want you be more determined to be successful in your life. These are things that anyone who really cares about people would want for you. You can read all the books you want. You start studying your symptoms. "Oh, I got that." "I got that." You start imagining sickness. Your mind is very, very powerful.

There were cases of false pregnancies. I don't know if you ever heard about it. A woman wants to have a baby. She can't get pregnant. She says to herself, *All my girlfriends are having babies. They are getting pregnant, but not me.* She lies in bed at night. She thinks about having a baby, and her stomach distends up to seven inches. Her breasts get larger, and milk forms. In the old days, doctors didn't have the technology we have today. The doctors treated these women for the whole nine months. At the end of the nine months, there is nothing there. The desire caused it to happen.

Do you know your mind can bring on sickness? You are worried about cancer. A package of cigarettes says it causes cancer. But people still smoke while looking at that message on the pack of cigarettes. There is more cancer than ever before. There is more diabetes than ever before, especially among children. I make sessions for children for bedwetting, proper food combining, losing weight, getting better grades in school, and stopping being a bully.

I want you to get benefits while you are reading this. You should read it more than once. When people listen to my sessions, they have to listen to them for a few months to get permanent results. But you get the results. The very first time you read this book, you are going to feel better. The very first time you hear the session, you are going to feel better. If you don't do it repetitively; it's going to come back to you. Mothers didn't say clean the plate, eat your food just once. They did it about twenty thousand times over an eighteen-year-period. That concept is deeply seated in the back of the mind. You don't have to read this book for eighteen years. You have to read or listen for a few months. You have to read even this portion of the book a number of times to get lasting results. The first time you read this, you will feel immediate results for two or three hours. Then, the next time you read this book, it will last two or three days. Then, the next time you read it, it will last two or three weeks. The next time you read it, it will last a few months.

You need to wash the banks out in the back of the subconscious. You have trillions and trillions of brain cells that are like little cameras that pick up sounds, smells, and feelings. It's all recorded there. Everything you've done in your life is recorded in the back of your mind. If you have severe depression, an alcohol problem, or a drug or sex problem, you need to download that free evaluation and fill it out. Get into this program. You are going to get results just reading this portion of the book. I want you to think of the large muscles in your thighs becoming loose and limp. You've been all knotted up and tensed up. You people with high blood pressure, just reading this part of this book is going to help lower your blood pressure. You people with headaches or depression are going to feel better. The Bible has all the answers. Again, A [happy] cheerful heart is good medicine,' Proverbs 17:22 (NIB).

People who drink have problems. Solve their problems, and they don't have to drink anymore. There are a lot of organizations that have you go for alcoholism or drug addiction, and you get up in front of class and you say, "I'm an alcoholic." "I'm a pilot." "I'm an alcoholic." "I'm a movie actor." "I'm an alcoholic." "I'm a singer." It is a bunch of BS. It's reinforcing your problem. People with addictions have problems. Solve their problems, and they don't have to be addicted any longer. A happy heart does good, like medicine.

I had a lady come in, but she didn't want to enroll. Her husband said, "Hey, I've got to do something. The psychiatrist is giving her all kinds of medication; she's taking about seven different ones."

I told him, "I'm not a doctor. Don't come off of medication without getting permission from your doctor. I'm a minister; I work for the man upstairs. I work for God. God didn't make any junk."

They came back in a few months. I didn't even know his wife. Her eyes were shining. They looked like big brown olives. She had a big smile on her face. She said, "I've not been happy since I was a little girl. What magic do you have in your sessions? I can't wait to get home to listen to them."

See, you don't have to listen for years. You have to read or listen for at least three months if you want to knock out alcohol, depression, or a sex problem. You need the repetition. But the thing is to find the reason you have depression. Find the reason you have a sex problem. Sometimes, sex is made dirty. It can work either way. Some people who have been sexually abused have a sex addiction. They want more. But other people don't want to be bothered. I find the root of the problem when you fill out the evaluation. We evaluate the form and use a computer to pinpoint the areas in which people need help.

I want to give you some suggestions. I don't want any mothers to think I am picking on them. You should honor thy father and honor thy mother. If you have some problems, it could be because of abuse while growing up. This isn't so in every case, but it is a causative factor in about 80 percent of the cases. How do you like that? That's a big number. So many women come to me that have been sexually abused by their stepfathers, fathers, grandfathers, and neighbors ... whatever. It ruins their lives. We can fix that. That is what God wants for you.

If you start a business or get a job and are doing well, and then, all of a sudden, you sabotage yourself and fall backward, you have a mental block. Let's find the mental block. Here are the suggestions. You are going to smile more. You are going to feel happier. If you have a weight problem, a small amount of food will be sufficient. It will make you feel full. When you look at the food, it will turn you off. When you see or hear the refrigerator door opening and closing, you won't think of food. As you watch people eat, you'll feel full.

These are only suggestions. I zero in on one subject at a time. Here, I'm trying to give you the general idea of how powerful God is. How powerful you are. It doesn't matter what your education level is. It doesn't matter your color. It doesn't matter. You can achieve success. You can do anything and everything you really want to do—if you do what Einstein said. The imagination is more powerful than knowledge. Knowledge will claim you didn't get enough school. You didn't do this. You didn't do that. If you can imagine success, you can be successful at anything you want to do. And just by reading these words, I want you to feel a difference in your body. You're going to stand straight. Your eyes are going to sparkle. You are going to feel happy. You are going to smile more. You are going to enjoy life more. If you work, you're going to enjoy your job more, no matter what the job is and even if you didn't like it before. Keep telling yourself, "I love my work, I love my work, I love my work." You are lucky you are working. A lot of people don't even have a job. See yourself programming yourself to be successful.

Now, when you are through reading this chapter and you stand up, you are going to feel the energy flow in your body. You will be wide-awake and alert, unless you want to crawl into bed and go to sleep. Then, you can go to sleep and sleep like a baby. People who have had insomnia or sleeping problems are going to find it is a lot easier to rest. You know why? Because you have found something that really works, and that's you. You have the power to change your lifestyle and to enjoy everything God has planned for you. If you're reading this, maybe God wanted you to pick up this book and read it. Maybe someone who loves you gave it to you as a gift, or you bought it yourself, or you want to buy copies for your loved ones. What goes around comes around. God bless you.

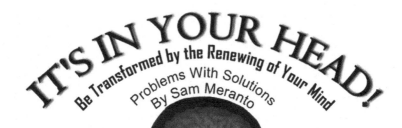

IT'S IN YOUR HEAD!
Be Transformed by the Renewing of Your Mind
Problems With Solutions
By Sam Meranto

WEIGHT LOSS
You can exercise and diet for years and the weight usually comes back plus additional pounds. the only way you can have permanent results is to de-program your subconscious mind from childhood training.

STRESS
Children, relationships, marital problems, childhood traumas, work, problems, are all straws that can break the camel's back and cause high blood pressure, strokes, heart attacks and many other physical problems. Sam de-programs these stressful problems with simple techniques he has developed over the last 30 years and thousands have gotten documented results

DRUGS
You try drugs because all yoour friends are do doing it - you know it's wrong, but after you use them a number of times, your subconscious becomes programmed and you have lost conscious control. Sam's help gives the control back to you! The same holds true for prescription drug dependency.

PAIN
Pain is your friend! It tells you to get that attention you can be taught to control the pain without medication

HEADACHES
Trace back to the first headache and find the underlying cause

MONEY
You may be "programmed to fail" from early childhood experiences by others who failed or who were content to be "just average". Sam erases your "failure programming" and reprograms a positive future for success.

SMOKING
Trace back to the first cigarette and find out what it represents. That is the key to permanent results.

SEXUAL PROBLEMS
Trace back to the first bad experience, even if it is buried deep in the subconscious, and eliminate it from your computer

MENTAL HEALTH
Caused by chemical imbalances in the brain. trace to traumatic experiences that caused the mind to stop producing God's natural chemicals deprogram bad experiences and reprogram with positive thinking.

CHILD ABUSE
Results from bad childhood experiences that you have received. De-program your childhood and turn the negatives into positives.

ALCOHOLISM
Most cases trace to parents, grandparents, and down the family tree. Eliminate the environmental experiences from the subconscious and this takes away the desire for alcohol.

TEMPERS
trace to early childhood experiences of others who had tempers and erase that negative programming from the subconsious mind.

SHYNESS & CONFIDENCE
Trace back to negaive suggestions given you to you by parents or teachers. find the cause, de-program it.

All Faith Self Help Center, Inc.
4440 E. Indian School Rd. Phoenix, AZ. 85018 602.957.4697

It's in Your Head

I want you to understand how powerful the subconscious mind is so I want to repeat this as stated in the last chapter. The average person retains very little of what they read or hear. That is why I'm repeating this information. It is very important and you should read this book a few times, not just once. The chapter "Read and trance away your problems" is the first time as far as our knowledge that anyone has ever put a person in a trance while reading. Although there is such a thing as road hypnosis where people stare at the center of the road and put themselves in a trance and accidents have occurred. But your reading the book in perfect safety. You don't have to worry about going off the road. Just like Sam made sessions that you can listen to to keep you awake while driving. This method can actually save many lives (truck drivers especially can benefit from this). It was developed by Sam in 1950 by working with deaf adults holding up scroll cards, which put them in a trance.

You can become a dietitian, a nurse, or even a doctor. You can know about all the proper foods to eat, and you can still eat wrong due to the eighteen years of being programmed to eat your food. If it took two years to program you not to roll out of the bed, and that stays with you for life, just imagine what eighteen years of, "Clean your plate; people are starving in Ethiopia," has done to you. It takes an act of God and a miracle to change what your loved ones have programmed you to do. According to the US government, the only way for permanent weight loss is to change your lifestyle. Sam will go on record, saying his program is the best in the world. His program is totally about lifestyle changes.

Sam was born November 3, 1931. At age twenty, he weighed 180 pounds. Today, sixty years later, Sam weighs 165 pounds. Actions speak louder than words. Sam still lifts barbells, takes his wife dancing—and I hate to admit this, but he dances a storm around me. I can't keep up with him … yet! He can paint or roof a house and do the same things he did when he was younger. Sam said, "I believe longevity has a lot to do with the way you think and the way you eat. A lot of people say it's in the genes."

One day Sam decided to get up on a ladder to touch up some paint. The ladder slipped out from under him, and he went down in a heap. He dislocated his right shoulder, ripped open his nose, and nearly lost his eye.

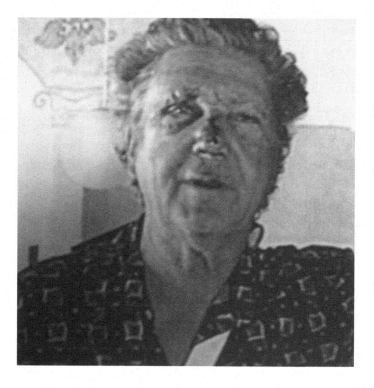

They had to put nine titanium pins in his right shoulder, because he had torn three muscles off of it. After spending over $4,300 at the Mayo Clinic, can you believe they actually missed diagnosing the damage to his shoulder—the reason Sam went to Mayo in the first place?

Patient's Name	Mayo Clinic Number	Visit Number	Dates of Service
MR. SAM R. MERANTO	6-927-395	8119	04/28/08-04/28/08

Please refer to patient's name, Mayo Clinic number and visit number on all correspondence.

THIS IS NOT A BILL - PLEASE RETAIN FOR YOUR RECORDS

Date of Service	Service Code	Service Description	Amount
04/28/08	08180051	ELECTROLYTE PANEL	97.00
04/28/08	08183204	CREATININE, (FOR-CT,IVP,HEMO)	27.00
04/28/08	08183215	GLUCOSE(S)	.00
04/28/08	08194520	UREA NITROGEN; QUANTITATIVE *	20.00
04/28/08	08109109	CBC W/5-PART WBC DIFFERENTL	50.00
04/28/08	08109236	PROTHROMBIN TIME	31.00
04/28/08	08185730	APTT	47.00
04/28/08	08109308	URINALYSIS, BY DIPSTICK	26.00
04/28/08	08170435	RD SHOULDER 2 VIEWS RIGHT	122.17
04/28/08	08172121	RD ED CHEST PA & LATERAL	128.80
04/28/08	08170486	CT MAXILLOFACIAL SCAN,W/O CONT	1,082.20
04/28/08	08172192	CT SCAN PELVIS W/O CONTRAST	1,122.37
04/28/08	08174150	CT ABDOMEN W/O CONTRAST	1,086.81
04/28/08	10081144	ED-FAC INTERMEDIATE III W/PROC	549.00
		TOTAL CHARGES	4,389.35

Once the problem was found, Sam was told he would never be able to lift his arm above his head again or lift weights. They were wrong! Today, because of Sam walking his talk, he is strong, healthy, and totally healed. Sam has full use of his arm and continues to lift weights to this day. Sam's program has been used by celebrities, athletes, and ordinary people.

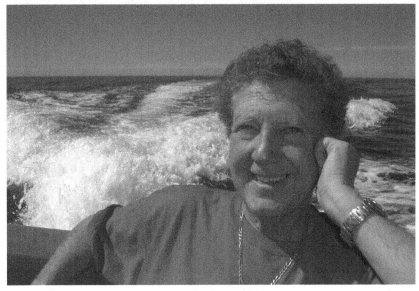

Sam today, healthy and happy.

If you buy a brand-new Rolls Royce, you should be able to agree with me that Rolls Royce has an *incredible* pedigree. They are considered one of the finest automobiles made today. Put some dirt in the oil and dirty gas in the tank, and you can say good-bye to the good genes it started out with. If you take after your relatives, being overweight and sickly, could it be you picked up their bad eating habits, and that's the real problem? Hispanics, African Americans, and Native Americans have the highest rate of diabetes and obesity. Could it be because of their culture and the way they eat? You don't have to be a rocket scientist to figure out that one. The only way to help them is to change their lifestyle and ask God to help.

When you build a house, you put in cement footing and then a concrete slab or cellar. You build it out of rebar and cement. If the contractor is trying to save money, he cuts back on the thickness of the cement and builds a beautiful house, putting the money where people can see it: stucco, tile roof, and granite countertops. But the foundation is weak. In the walls, lurks particleboard made of wood chips, glue, and bad chemicals. Eventually, the foundation will start to crack, and the beautiful house will start to fall apart.

Humans are like a house. If they don't have a good foundation that starts in the mothers' womb, as time goes on, they start to fall apart with physical and psychological problems. Sam goes to the root of the issues fast and then makes sessions for these problems. Sam calls himself "Contractor Sam," building a new foundation in your mind.

Sam offered to help the state of Arizona save millions of dollars by donating his program for free in the Arizona state mental hospitals. During this time of economic crisis, those funds could be better spent on other vital issues. On the following pages is a copy of his letter to Governor Jan Brewer and the response. Sadly, she probably never even saw the letter, and the response Sam received indicated no interest in considering such a generous offer.

Governor Jan Brewer Mental illness is on the rise costing Arizona millions of dollars.
You do not have to appropriate more money for drugs.

July 30, 2010

Honorable Governor Jan Brewer:

You got what it takes to make things happen to improve our state and I compliment you for having the determination to succeed. I would like to put my program into the States mental institutions. I have licensed M.D.'s on our staff to help supervise. I will do the test for free to prove we can save millions of dollars and help the poor souls being drugged out of their minds.

Psychiatry and Psychology's track record is very poor. According to psychiatrist Jim Norris M.D. said he learned more in two weeks on my program than all his 30 years in practice and medical training combined. I have his testimonial on video, copy enclosed. Take the time to look at it. He also said that all he did was rely on medication to alter people's minds. You took the bull by the tail when you took on the illegal immigration problem. Now you are going to have to take your psychiatry department by the tail. They don't want to try my program, because they are afraid of losing their jobs. Some of them are dedicated men and women that are open minded to new ideas and I would gladly work with them. But I am more concerned about saving the State millions of dollars and helping the poor souls that are in desperate need. If you would give me the contract for mental health or put me in charge of supervising your treatment centers. I guarantee better results and I'll save the state money. If I can't deliver you pay me nothing. Don't be concerned by how many degrees I have. Be concerned about how many people that I have helped here in Phoenix in the last 35 years at the same address.

I have been teaching psychiatrists, psychologists, and professors my technique in Boston, Ma. since 1952. I am self educated and a pioneer in mental health. I would love to hear from you. May God bless you and guide you in everything you undertake.

All Faith Self Help Center - 4440 E. Indian School Rd. - Phoenix, AZ 85018
602-957-4697 - 1-800-580-5080

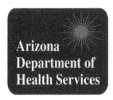

Office of the Director

150 N. 18th Avenue, Suite 500
Phoenix, Arizona 85007-3247
(602) 542-1025
(602) 542-1062 FAX
Internet: www.azdhs.gov

JANICE K. BREWER, GOVERNOR
WILL HUMBLE, DIRECTOR

August 24, 2010

Sam Meranto
All Faith Self Help Center
4440 East Indian School Road
Phoenix, Arizona 85018

Dear Mr. Merento:

I am writing on behalf of Governor Brewer in response to the informational disc in which was sent to her, and received on August 6, 2010.

Thank you very much for the disc however, the Department of Health Services currently does not offer spiritual/religious counseling. In order for you to be considered for any state contract you will have to visit the Arizona Department of Administration, State Procurement Office website at http//www.spo.az.gov/. There you will find a wealth of information pertaining to doing business with the State of Arizona, how to become a state vendor as well as becoming notified of any state solicitations.

Again, thank you for the information as it is much appreciated.

Sincerely,

Will Humble
Director

WH:sb

Leadership for a Healthy Arizona

40

Longevity has a lot to do with the way you think and the way you eat.

Sam Meranto

Fruit, Roots, and Hearts

The All Faith Self-Help Center Sam founded is a church organization unlike any other church in the world. Churches pray for you when you are sick or in the hospital and after you die. Sam's church prays for you while you are alive. The church does everything possible to keep you out of the hospital for as long as possible by teaching you the proper way to eat and to control depression, pain, smoking, drugs, and alcohol.

Most sicknesses start in the mind and in the digestive system. Most churches have fellowship, where church members are asked to bring their favorite foods, pies, cakes, and things that cause obesity and sickness. It is written in the Bible that being a glutton is a sin. All the instructions on how to eat are in the Bible.

When God made the world, he made plants, trees, and the fruit they bear as food. He gave animals the same. According to the Old Testament, the average life span was two hundred fifty years. They did not eat meat. After the great flood, there was no more plant life, so God blessed the animals and said it was okay to eat them. The average life span of a man dropped to twenty-five to thirty years old. Sam is not telling you not to eat meat … but to eat less of it. He designed a program called "Fruits, Roots, and Hearts." You will not make it to 250, but according to medical science, you could make it to over 125 without being in a wheelchair.

Sam's church teaches you how to eat and control depression without medication. I repeat: the Bible states, "A [happy] cheerful heart is good medicine,' Proverbs 17:22 (NIB). Man-made medicine can cause severe side effects and suicidal tendencies. For temporary use, it has its benefits, so always follow your doctor's advice. But get a doctor who believes in

43

God and the power of the mind. If you have doctors who don't believe this, fire them and get ones who do.

All these problems can be solved very easily without mind-altering drugs. The United States is the greatest country in the world, but in my opinion, it is so backward when it comes to mind control. In Sam's opinion the medical profession prescribes more drugs in this country than in all the other countries in the world combined. No wonder drug pushers come to our country: it's a ready-made market. The United States is conditioned by the medical profession to rely on drugs for every ache and pain. They even prescribe drugs to children as young as two years old for hyperactivity!

Dr. Walter J. Freeman II became the father of Lobotomies in America. His partner, Egas Moniz, won the widely criticized "Nobel Prize" in 1959 for discovering the lobotomy. It was used to treat mental illness. He is credited for developing the transorbital—ice pick—lobotomy. Dr. Freeman performed over twenty-nine hundred lobotomies during his career, including the first prefrontal lobotomy in the United States. Some of his patients were as young as four. They were given lobotomies because they were hyperactive and hard to handle. The lobotomy put them in an easy to handle, zombie-like state. He would take an instrument similar to an ice pick and insert it into the corner of one or both eye sockets. He would move it around, until connections to the prefrontal cortex were severed.

Some kids of that time were told by their parents if they didn't behave, they would be taken to Dr. Freeman. Actress Francis Farmer, at age thirty-eight became hysterical and couldn't handle her affairs and money. Her mother had her power of attorney and put her in an asylum. She allowed the doctors to perform a lobotomy. Her mother then took over Francis's affairs. Francis spent the rest of her life in a controllable state. We've been trained to look up to our doctors and clergy and now we all know what a big mistake that can be. Most of us have loving, caring mothers, but they had faith in their doctors. In those days, they didn't have the mind-altering drugs we have today that replaced the lobotomy.

I could not write a book without bringing up Sam's incredible wife, Cynthia. She is as beautiful inside as she is outside. They have been married for almost thirty years, and in today's world, that alone speaks volumes. Sam first met Cynthia in 1979, when she came to work for him. Out of curiosity about what Sam was up to, she started listening to his sessions. She had problems and issues about being adopted and like most young people she drank and smoked. Cynthia also had issues with weight and ended up losing twenty pounds, stopped drinking and smoking! What is so powerful is that Sam's program teaches you how to keep the weight off for life and today, after 30 years Cynthia still weights 124 pounds. So, not only was she able to shed weight, she has been able to maintain the weight loss for over thirty-two years without depriving herself of any food. Again, actions speak louder than words, and Sam was stating the need to do a lifestyle change as the answer to avoiding obesity over three decades ago!

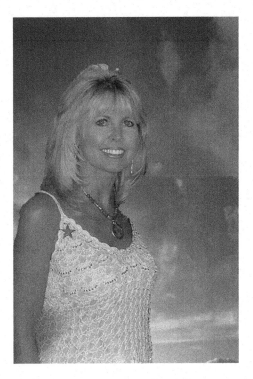

A [happy] cheerful heart is good medicine.

Proverbs 17:22 (NIB)

Children Are Our Future

Children have been given mind-altering drugs that have caused severe physical and psychological problems and suicide. The young man who killed over thirty students and himself at Virginia Tech had a history of taking mind-altering drugs prescribed to him by doctors. In my opinion, because he was picked on and bullied most of his life he became depressed, and the medication made him suicidal. He knew he was going to kill himself, so he decided to take some of the bullies with him plus some innocent bystanders.

A dear friend of mine was murdered by her husband in Utah a few years ago, and her husband blamed this outrageous behavior on mind-altering drugs. Today, these stories seem to happen far too often. Something drastic needs to be done to stop this behavior before the lives of others are taken. I truly believe Sam's program is the answer.

The sessions that Sam makes talk about drugs, smoking, and bullying to stop them at the source. Sam knows firsthand what it is like to be bullied. As a twelve-year-old kid, Sam had a bully come after him with an ice pick in the school yard. Someone yelled out, "Watch out for Whitey. He has an ice pick." God was with Sam. With his left hand, Sam was able to grab Whitey's arm with the ice pick in it and punched him with his right, breaking his nose.

The principal took them to the school basement and said to both of them, "Go ahead. Continue the fight or shake hands."

Whitey said, "I'm bleeding. I quit. Let's shake hands." And Sam and Whitney became friends. God was with Sam. Today, it is so much scarier, since kids carry guns!

In Sam's sessions, he works with kids to stop fighting. However, in extreme cases, they must be strong enough to defend themselves. Most bullies are abused by other people, and some by their own parents. When they go to school, they pick on weaker, defenseless people to get out their frustrations of being abused by someone else.

Sam makes sessions to help young people be happy and more understanding of others. If you have any problems with a child, contact Sam's office. If you are having money problems Sam might give them to you for free; you just pay the postage. If you can afford to pay, that will allow Sam to help more who can't.

Sam & Children with disabilities

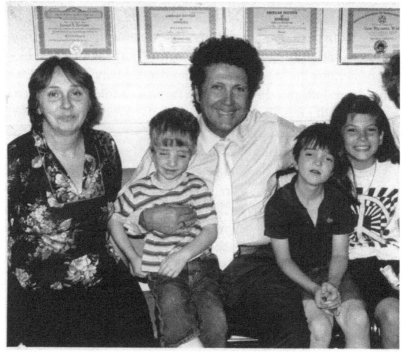

Mrs. Holtz brought her two grandson's to Sam.
They were born with a rare malady called Krohn's disease, they had difficulties functioning as normal pre-schoolers. Sam donated his sessions FREE for the two boys & her daughter seen in the far right.
Within one year the two boys were in regular kindergarten.
(which doctors said would never be poosible) Kathy the daughter won an Arizona championship for writing a poem called "Kathys Clown."
In this picture, the family came back to thank Sam for his help. © by Sam Meranto, 2008

We should do everything we can to protect our children, and we should all take an active part in doing so. There is an old saying, "Sticks and stones may break my bones, but words will never hurt me." That saying is wrong, because words (such as name-calling) *can* seriously harm you. Most people who are abused take it for a long period of time and then they snap. Sam lets bullies know they are putting themselves in danger when they pick on innocent, weak people. No matter how weak someone is, it only takes a tenth of a pound of pressure and a blink of an eye to get revenge. Sam's sessions have been successfully tested on many young people and helped them avoid physical and further emotional damage.

We should do everything we can to protect our children, and we should all take an active part in doing so.

Your Blueprint

A psychiatrist brought his son to Sam with a computer printout of what was wrong with him. He held the printed list up in the air and let it drop to the floor—he was 6'2"—and told Sam to read it. He said it was better to let someone else help his son than to do it himself, which happens to be true. Children will take advice from someone other than their parents. His son was twenty-two years old. While watching television at home, his father said he would jump up and start yelling in the middle of a program. And he was failing miserably in school.

None of the things on the printed list had anything to do with his son's problems. Sam worked with him for half a day. He told the son he would not tell his father anything he said, because he was of legal age and had a right to his privacy. But Sam also told him that since his father was a licensed doctor, it was okay for him to give his dad the information. Sam said, "If you don't follow my instructions, I will tell your dad what the problem is!" Of course, Sam was just bluffing, because legally and ethically, he could not and would not give the father any information. But Sam's bluff worked. The son was afraid his father would find out what he was doing and followed the program.

Now, here was his problem. The young man stopped at an adult bookstore. A guy who worked there talked to him about homosexuality. He got him smoking pot and watching X-rated movies. Eventually, they started doing homosexual acts with each other. He was a Christian, so Sam asked him to ask God for forgiveness, with Sam as his witness. He was absolved of his sins and became a born-again Christian. That was fifteen years ago, and the young man is now a medical doctor.

Sam does not infringe on anyone's religious beliefs, but he does talk about God to everyone. He calls on the Holy Spirit for the Jewish faith and all other religions that don't believe Jesus Christ was their savior, as they all do believe in a Holy Spirit.

This twenty-two year old followed Sam's instructions and came back to see him a year later. He had become an "A" student, cleaned up his act, and had a part time job. He said, "God must have sent me to you." He believes in God more than ever before.

As mentioned earlier, Sam has everyone fill out a Lifestyle Analysis of 225 specialized questions. The questionnaire is then used to pinpoint the areas in which you need help. Then, his staff goes to Sam's library of over seventeen hundred prerecorded sessions and hand selects the sessions right for you—no matter what the subject. Each program is personalized for the individual. There is nothing like this in the world. It is the strongest, most effective program you can imagine, and again, I speak firsthand as a successful client of Sam's program. Once you fill out the evaluation, you can use the CDs in the program to BE WHAT YOU WANT TO BE.

Albert Einstein said, "The imagination is more powerful than knowledge." (By Rodger Constandse, ezinearticle.com). Knowledge will tell you that you have a problem, but the imagination can override it! Many people have cured themselves of cancer and other diseases by imagining good health and praying to God for help (Reader's Digest May 2001 "The healing power of faith" by Lydia Strohl and Good Housekeeping November 1997 "Think yourself well by Martha Barnette). So, if you need help or know someone who does, check out Sam's program at www.sammeranto.com or call 1-800-580-5080.

The imagination is more powerful than knowledge.

Albert Einstein

A Miracle for You

In my opinion, actions always speak louder than words. Sam could not still be in business today, after fifty years (thirty six years at the same location in Phoenix) if these stories were not true.

Many dedicated men, women—some medical doctors—refer clients to Sam and believe in the power of faith. His sessions have been used at both Yale Hospital in New Haven, Connecticut, and at Tucson Medical Center for severe pain and depression. Sam thanks the medical doctors who believe in the Hippocratic Oath they took to do everything in their power to help and heal their patients.

People will spend more money on a vacation that has no lasting effects than they will on a program to make them healthy, happy, and prosperous. Imagine the positive effect such a program could have for you and for generations to come.

The following stories and pictures will help you understand why I am so excited to share Sam with you. His affect on people for the last fifty plus years is amazing. These are just a handful of the numerous stories Sam has to share. We have been given permission to use all of the names and pictures contained in this book by the people themselves.

Sam is a self-educated man, doing the seemingly impossible. When doctors, hospitals, psychologists, psychiatrists, and even faith healers were unable to help, Sam was able to find the problems in minutes. Sam firmly believes in the power of the mind and that God has changed these people.

Today, Sam enjoys donating sessions to hospitals, children centers, and correctional institutions. His sessions have been sent to the motion picture industry, where Sam has had the opportunity to meet many of the stars over the years.

As mentioned earlier, if you need help or know someone who does, call 1-800-580-5080, or go to www.sammeranto.com and download the free evaluation form. Get enrolled in this life-changing program and begin your healing process.

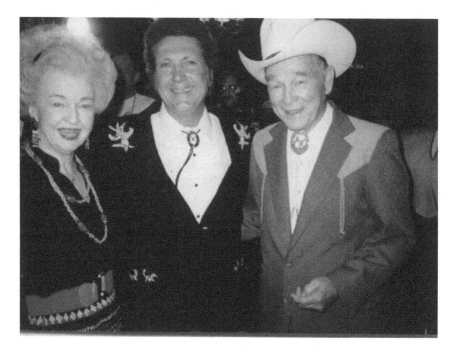

THREE HUNDRED FIFTY-POUND WEIGHT LOSS

350 Pound Weight Loss

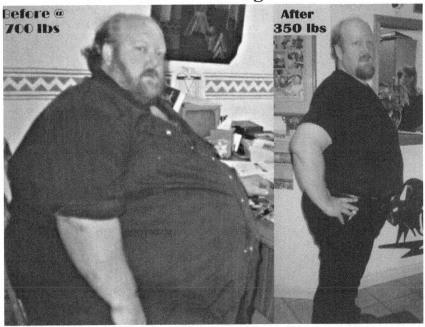

Before @ 700 lbs

After 350 lbs

Mike came to Sam's office weighing in at approximately seven hundred pounds. The office scale only went up to five hundred pounds, so they used two scales and had him put a foot on each scale. He said he had tried every diet possible and then had his stomach stapled. He lost two hundred pounds, but all the weight slowly came back. He tried Sam's program out of desperation.

He came back to see Sam a year and half later, after he lost three hundred and fifty pounds. You can see the incredible change in the pictures. In his words, "You saved my life."

Sam said, "Thank God for giving me the gift to help you."

RHEUMATIC HEART DISEASE

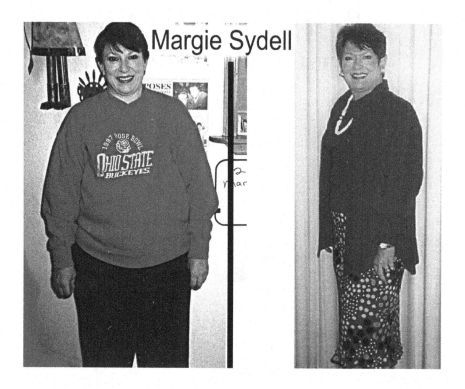

Margie Sydell

Margie Sydell had rheumatic heart disease for thirty-eight years. She had five heart surgeries, a stroke, congestive heart failure, and diabetes. After coming in to see Sam at his All Faith Self-Help Center, she was able to reduce her glucose readings, lost thirty pounds, and now feels like a new woman. She smiles all the time and feels like she has a chance to live again.

BROKEN BACK

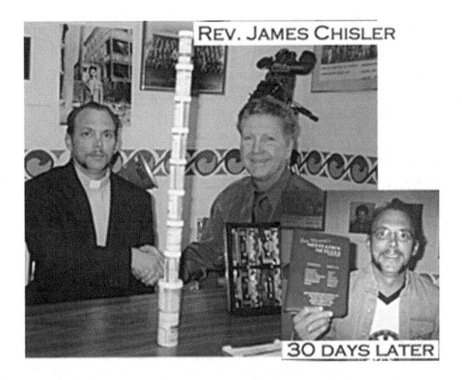

REV. JAMES CHISLER

30 DAYS LATER

Reverend Chisler was a champion bull rider. One day, a bull ended up on top of him and broke his back. When he came to Sam, he was on twenty-one prescriptions and hooked on painkillers.

After one month of using Sam's program, Reverend Chisler was able to cut his prescriptions down to only three. Here is his doctor's note, stating the reduction.

PUEBLO FAMILY PHYSICIANS, LTD.
DON G. CUNNINGHAM, D.O.
DEA # AC 1262194
DOUGLAS L. CUNNINGHAM, D.O.
DEA # BC 0956384
SHERRI L. SESSLER, PA-C
DEA # MS 0420555
DAWN K. DUFF, PA-C
DEA # MK 0591328
JUDITH BERGMAN, F.N.P.
DEA # MB 0585818
PATRIC HERNANDEZ-KLINE, F.N.P., M.S.N.
DEA # MH 0815867
4350 N. 19TH AVENUE, SUITE 6
PHOENIX, AZ 85015
(602) 264-9191 TEL. (602) 274-7184 FAX

NAME _James Chisler_

AGE _____

ADDRESS _____

DATE _12-10-7_

Rx ILLEGAL IF NOT SAFETY BLUE BACKGROUND

℞

Pt is doing well re. Back pain - he may use _less_ medication which is great. His MS has been ↓ to 40g BID.

Refill _____ times

DISPENSE AS WRITTEN

SUBSTITUTION PERMISSIBLE

3IFP0228189

OVER ONE HUNDRED POUNDS LOST

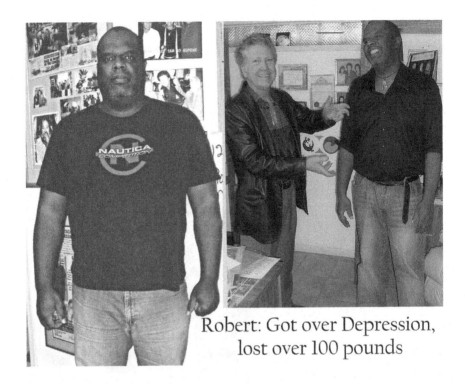

Robert: Got over Depression,
lost over 100 pounds

After losing over one hundred pounds, Robert had better self-worth and more energy to do a better job at work. This got him a promotion and a raise!

FROM DEPRESSION TO HAPPINESS IN SIX MINUTES!

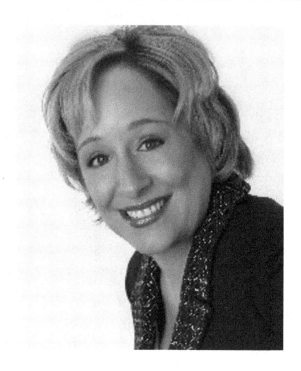

An unexpected change in my industry changed my life overnight. Years of hard work and commitment were gone in an instant. I was blindsided. Without Sam's program I would have taken it a lot harder and sunk into a serious depression. Instead, I am happy and loving life! Like Sam says, God made the world in six days, so why should it take years to fix our problems? Sam found my issues in six minutes and then he gave me a personalized program to fix the problem. I've been to many doctors and places and none of them had the answers or helped me. Sam truly has a gift from God, this is something that can't be learned in school – it's a natural gift from above. I truly believe everyone can benefit from Sam!

NEW LEG AND DRUG FREE

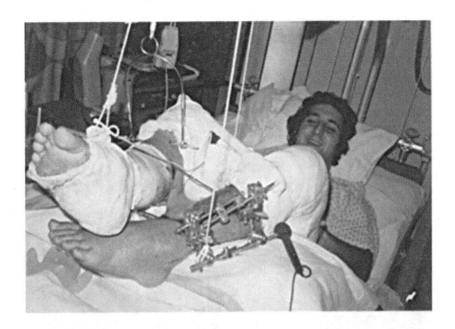

PROGRESS RECORD

TUCSON MEDICAL CENTER
PHYSICIAN'S PROGRESS NOTES

Dear Ms Mercato
Thanks very much for your help
with Tim. The motivational
tapes have helped him a great deal
to cope psychologically with his injury

Sincerely,
Jim Collins, M.D.

In 1983, Tim Klatt went to Mexico to have some fun on his motorcycle and was hit by a truck. He lay on the side of the road for three hours before help arrived. Tucson Medical Center sent an ambulance to pick him up, but on the way back to Tucson, the ambulance ran out of gas!

It took quite a bit of time to get the seriously injured Tim to the hospital. His left calf had been stripped to the bone of skin and muscle. The calf muscle was hanging loose. He was bleeding profusely.

Tim's sister Dee Gilenwater had come to Sam's office to lose weight some time before his accident. She successfully released forty pounds and was sold on Sam's program. After Tim's accident, she came to Sam and asked if there was anything he could do to help her brother. She was worried he was going to become a drug addict because of all the morphine he was being given. She said that at one point, Tim grabbed a nurse by the throat and begged for more morphine. He was becoming violent.

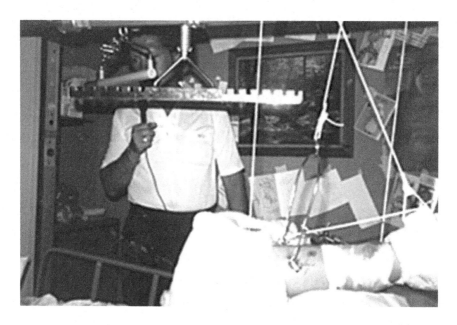

Sam immediately took out his recorder and made a personal tape for Tim to listen to while he was in the hospital. His sister introduced Sam to her brother on the recorded session and took it to him in the hospital. He threw the tape at the wall saying, "The hospital had me listen to tapes, and they don't work."

Dee said, "Sam is different. Just try it." So, he did. From that point on, Tim never took another shot of morphine. The doctors took a piece of the muscle from his right leg and attached it to the bone of the left leg. On the recorded session, Sam had him visualize that the blood was circulating, and the leg muscle was growing, growing, growing. Dr. Collins called Sam to tell him about the miracle: *Tim actually grew a new leg!*

The nurses played the tape every hour on the hour. Then, can you believe this? Someone actually stole the tape deck with the tape in it. Dr. Collins called Sam, begging him to come to the hospital. Sam's wife brought an 8mm movie camera with her, and they recorded the session in the hospital. The rest is history. Twenty-five years have gone by, and Tim is running and jogging today.

The Associated Press found out about Tim's miracle and ran a story titled, "Phoenix Man Has Found a Way to Cure Many Ills."

They misquoted Sam as saying, "Most psychiatrists and psychologists should be put in jail because of the result of their treatments" (although that statement has *some* validity). In some countries, if a doctor misdiagnoses you with a mental illness, it is a felony. In the United States, there is no punishment for making mistakes. That is why they call it a practice!

Tucson&Arizona

Monday, June 27, 1983

Think Faith Center Inc.
4440 E. Broadway School
Phoenix, AZ 85018
(602) 333-4867 or 45508

Tucson Citizen C

Phoenix hypnotist says he has the way to cure many ills

By JAMES E. WALTERS

PHOENIX — Hypnotist Jim Meramo says

PSYCHIATRIST LOSES LICENSE

Sam once had a client who was a psychiatrist and hooked on cocaine. He admitted he was so stoned out of his mind that he would diagnose people with bipolar disorder, schizophrenia, or whatever came to mind! The harm done to these people is outrageous and inexcusable. The public has been trained by their parents, and society, to trust their doctor. People believe the labels their doctors place on them! Even if they don't have the problem, they start reading books about the supposed problem and start imagining that they really have the problem. Sam worked with this psychiatrist personally, got him off the cocaine, found out about some childhood problems that caused him to have deep seated problems. He got his license back and became the top psychiatrist at one of the biggest psychiatric hospitals in the world eighteen years ago. I am not using his name to protect his identity.

Dan Haggerty, star of the television series *The Life and Times of Grizzly Adams,* was in a motorcycle accident, too, and had heard about Tim's story. You'll read about his story next.

DAN HAGGARTY: STAR OF THE LIFE AND TIMES OF GRIZZLY ADAMS

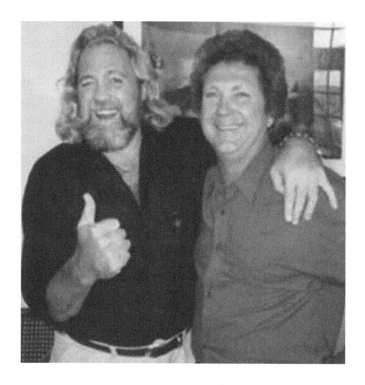

Dan had heard about Tim's story. He also ended up in a motorcycle accident. The blood would not circulate to his toes. Sam sent Dan a tape specifically for him.

This photo is of Dan thanking Sam for his help. Believe it or not, Dan still rides his motorcycle! Dan was so happy with the results from Sam's program that he came on Sam's TV infomercial that was played nationally on Discovery Channel and BET. In fact, Sam was recently featured on Discovery Channel's "Solutions to Your Problems," on the *Tree Hugger* series, giving hope to those watching and listening.

CHRONIC PAIN

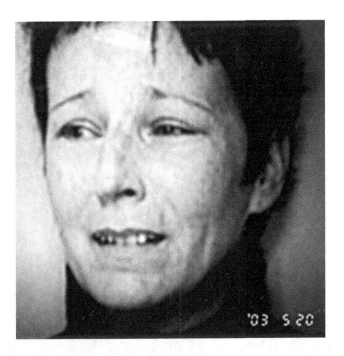

One day, Patty's husband brought her into Sam's center. She was in so much pain she could barely walk. She had to lie down on the chairs in the lobby. Patty had been rushed to the hospital every day for thirty days with panic attacks and severe headaches. Her husband lost his job and their house, because he had to take care of her and their eleven-year-old daughter.

He told Sam he doubted anyone could help his wife. Patty had seen over thirty doctors—psychiatrists, psychologists, and other PhDs and MDs. Sam told him he could have his wife feeling better by the time they left his office. Patty's husband said, "If it sounds too good to be true, it can't be true." He said they were broke. Their last trip was to a famous psychiatrist in Palm Springs, California, and it cost him all the money they had left. And it didn't help. In fact, she got more medication and felt worse. This is all on video in Sam's office.

Sam told him the center was a nonprofit organization, and he would work with Patty for free if he could record her getting well to help other people. Patty's husband said he would sign or do anything to get his wife well. Below, you can see the picture of Patty two weeks later, ready to go back to work as a hairdresser. Can you believe the change in her from the first picture?

Just imagine Patty being rushed to the emergency room every day for thirty days. Sam found the problem in six minutes. She left his office the first day feeling better. Patty said, "Sam is the fastest, most successful therapist that ever lived. He is a gift from God."

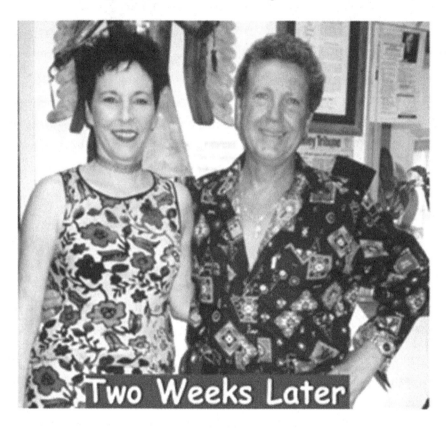

Two Weeks Later

If anyone is not getting satisfaction from hospitals and doctors, you can download the evaluation online to begin the process of enrolling in the program. Mail it into Sam's office at 4440 E. Indian School Road Phoenix, AZ 85018. You do not want your personal business on the internet. That is why the US mail is the best way or personally bring it into our office if you live nearby. They analyze your evaluation and pinpoint the problems that your having. Then they select from a specialized library of over seventeen hundred pre-recorded sessions to personalize your program. Individualizing the program for each person is part of the secret to his success.

Sessions can be sent anywhere in the world, so it is not necessary to come to Phoenix for help. Don't give up. Pray about it, and God will give you the answer. For more information, call 602-957-4669 or 1-800-580-5080.

SEVERE DEPRESSION: LOSS OF A LOVED ONE

Debbie was brought in by her mother and father, who were in their seventies. Her parents said that for some reason, she was mentioning Sam Meranto a lot. At wits end, Debbie parents, looked Sam up in the phone book.

She had seen over twenty-five doctors and been hospitalized on numerous occasions. She was very unkempt and had not bathed in who knows how long. She was delirious and kept saying Sam's name, even as her parents walked into Sam office. They had decided it was worth a try and enrolled her in Sam's program.

Sam made a session with her to take home and got a release to use the pictures and any videos to help people with depression. After all, seeing is believing.

Sam put her in a meditative state and asked her why she was repeating his name. She was grieving over the loss of her husband, who had died of lung cancer caused by smoking. For years, he kept telling her he wanted to go to Sam Meranto. He wanted to get help to quit smoking. She insisted he could do it on his own. After his death, she felt guilty. If only she had listened to her husband, he could still be alive—or so she thought.

While she was still in a meditative state, Sam told her that her husband is happy where he is and still loves her. He did not hold her responsible for his death. She reacted immediately, and after only two weeks, there was a drastic change for the better. This is obvious in the "after" picture.

Sam has sessions for those dealing with the loss of a loved one. I have benefited from these sessions, having lost my first son at ten weeks old from sudden infant death syndrome, my father unexpectedly at sixty-three, and my dear mother at seventy-three. I have had two close friends murdered.

The benefit from his sessions for the loss of a loved one is amazing: life altering. I don't know how I ever got by before Sam. I see things so differently now, and I am happy! If you know anyone who has lost a loved one, he or she will love his sessions. The pain from the loss of a loved one can come out in so many different areas in your life: weight gain, anger, and more. The benefits of resolving these issues can be huge and widespread. The issues can be resolved in a short time with money well spent.

Debbie - Depression & Anxieties
Before   After

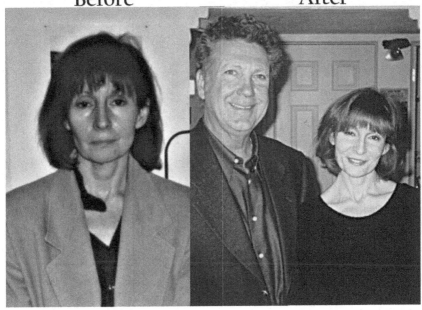

PARKINSON'S DISEASE:
Mary White Lost Weight
and Stopped Shaking

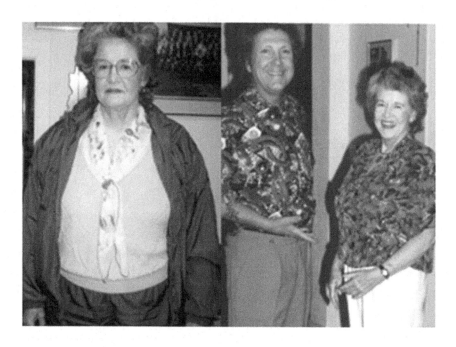

Mary came into Sam's office, shaking uncontrollably from Parkinson's. She was unable to go out to eat, because she couldn't hold onto the silverware. This caused her to be depressed. She wanted to lose some weight, as well. After listening to Sam's sessions, she was able to control her shaking and was able to go out to eat with her friends—without throwing food at them. She also lost almost forty pounds. Look at the difference in her pictures. She looks twenty years younger.

THREE WEEKS IN A COMA:
Fernando Mungia

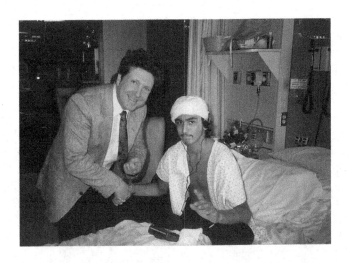

See Fernando, twenty years later, on the next page.
SIX KIDS, TWENTY YEARS LATER, THANKING SAM

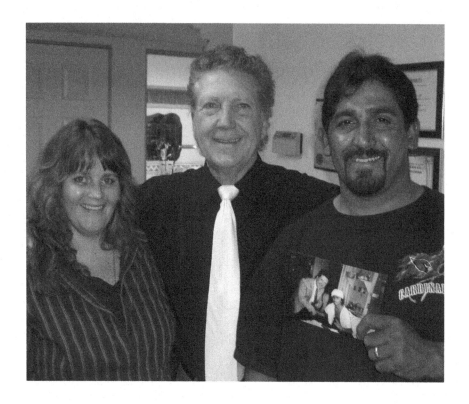

Fernando was in an automobile wreck and in a coma for three weeks when he was only seventeen years old. His girlfriend at the time came to Sam and asked for his help. She told Sam if Fernando did wake up, he would be in a vegetative state. The doctors said there was very little they could do; there was almost no hope that he would be normal if he did wake up.

Sam gave her a special recorded session telling him to wake up and he would remember everyone. After she played it four times, Fernando woke perfectly normal and remembered everyone. It was another miracle from God. She called and told Sam the good news. Sam went to the hospital and took photographs and a super 8 sound movie of the miracle. The second picture is from twenty years later, with Fernando and his family thanking Sam.

Sam has donated his sessions to many organizations and hospitals, such as Arizona Corrections, Yale Hospital, Desert Vista Hospital, and the Motion Picture Country Hospital.

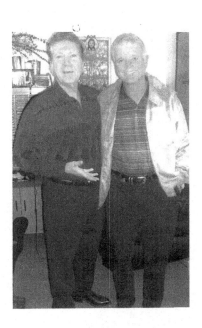

Jim Ahearn is a golf pro but never had a tournament win. When he came to Sam, he wanted to play a better round of golf. Sam made a session for playing better golf and told Jim he could be what he wanted to be. The result is shown below in a newspaper article showing $1.3million dollar win.

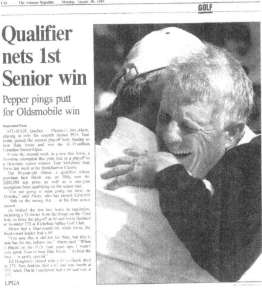

GOLF

Qualifier nets 1st Senior win

Pepper pings putt for Oldsmobile win

Associated Press

STE-JULIE, Quebec — Phoenix's Jim Ahern, playing in only his seventh Senior PGA Tour event, parred the second playoff hole Sunday to beat Hale Irwin and won the $1.35 million Canadian Senior Open.

It was the second week in a row that Irwin, a five-time champion this year, lost in a playoff to a first-time senior winner. Tom McGinnis beat Irwin last week at the BankBoston Classic.

The 50-year-old Ahern, a qualifier whose previous best finish was an 18th, won the $202,500 top prize as well as a one-year exemption from qualifying on the senior tour.

"I'm not going to miss going out there on Monday," said Ahern, who has earned $268,050 50th on the money list — in his first senior season.

He birdied the last two holes in regulation, including a 15-footer from the fringe on the 72nd hole, to force the playoff as he and Irwin finished at 16-under 272 at Richelieu Valley Golf Club. Ahern had a final round 68, while Irwin, the third-round leader, had a 69.

"I'm sorry this is old hat for Hale, but this is new hat for me, believe me," Ahern said. "When I played on the PGA Tour years ago, I wasn't very good. Now to beat Hale Irwin — to beat the best — is pretty special."

Ed Dougherty closed with a 67 to finish third at 273, Tom Jenkins shot a 67 and was fourth at 275, while David Lundstrom had a 69 and was at 275.

LPGA

BROKEN LEG AND
ABOUT TO LOSE JOB

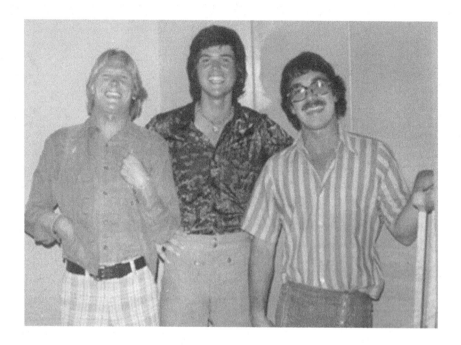

This is Donny Osmond in 1976, pictured here with the Rico brothers, who were jugglers. They were appearing in the *Donny and Marie Show* at the Hilton in Las Vegas. The one with the crutches broke his leg while playing volleyball. He is thanking Sam for having a special session with him to take away the pain and get him to go onstage with a cast on his foot. They were having trouble juggling flames *before* the accident, so Mr. Osmond, Donny's dad, was going to replace the Rico brothers with another act if they didn't improve.

Sam's son, Jeff, was playing volleyball with them on top of the Hilton. He told them his father could help Alex, the one with the broken foot, with his pain and juggling better than ever before. Jeff brought them over to where his dad was staying in Vegas and asked if he could help. The first thing Sam asked the Rico brothers was who they thought were the greatest jugglers in the world. They mentioned a few people.

Sam put both Rico brothers into a meditative state and told them they were now the world's greatest jugglers. Evidently they both believed it! In the show that evening, they juggled better than they ever had. Mr. Osmond was so impressed, he invited Jeff and Sam to have dinner with him after one of the shows. Mr. Osmond told Sam he decided to keep the Rico brothers in the show.

Thirty-two years passed, and Sam met up with Donny again. He didn't remember Sam at first; after all, that was over three decades ago. But as soon as Sam mentioned the Rico brothers playing volleyball at the top of the Hilton and how one broke his leg, that was all he had to say. Like a flash, Donny's memory came back, and he said, "How have you been all these years?" Look at the picture, which Donny autographed with, "Great to see you again."

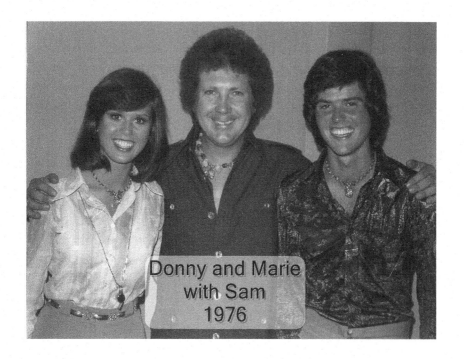

Donny and Marie
with Sam
1976

Here is a photograph of Marie and Donny. The
one below was taken thirty-two years later.

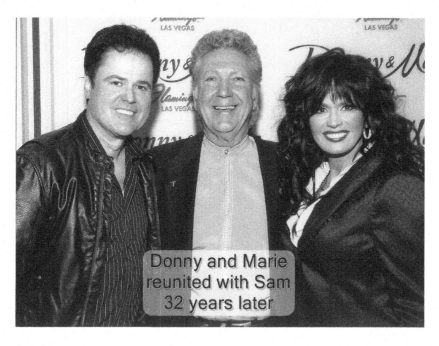

Donny and Marie
reunited with Sam
32 years later

DONNY OSMOND REMEMBERED SAM AFTER 32 YEARS!
No one remembers somone after 32 years! See what Donny wrote.

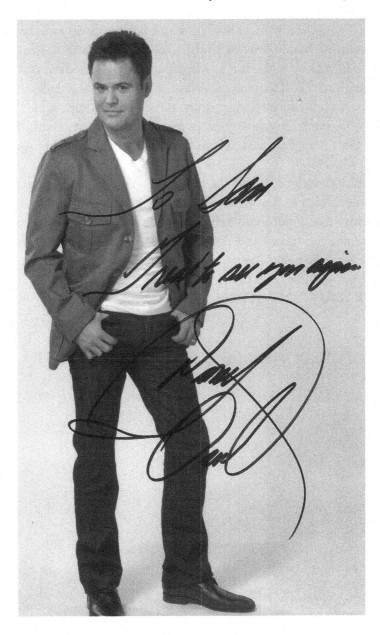

Sam first met Donny and Marie and the whole family backstage decades ago. He said they were one of the nicest families he ever met. Donny told Sam about his first car, which was given to him by General Motors. Sam got to witness firsthand how Mr. Osmond ran the show. He taught his family how to study, practice, and be successful. Sam admired how close Marie was to her dad and how she looked up to and respected him. Most women try to find a man like their dads.

Sam is a self-educated man, doing the seemingly impossible. When doctors, hospitals, psychologists, psychiatrists, and even faith healers were unable help, Sam was able to find the problems in minutes. This is a gift from God.

Sam has helped hospitals, children centers, and correctional institutions. He has sent tapes to the motion picture industry and has met many stars. If you need help or know someone who does, you can go to sammeranto.com and download the "Lifestyle Evaluation." Fill out the form to begin the process of enrolling in his program. Why waste years on programs that don't get to the issue, when you can BE WHAT YOU WANT TO BE?

Sam is the fastest, most successful therapist that ever lived. He is a gift from God.

Patty Cramer

10-day program at a

BEAUTIFUL RESORT NEAR PRESCOTT

for drug and alcohol abuse is available for less than half the cost of most alternative programs, and with better results!

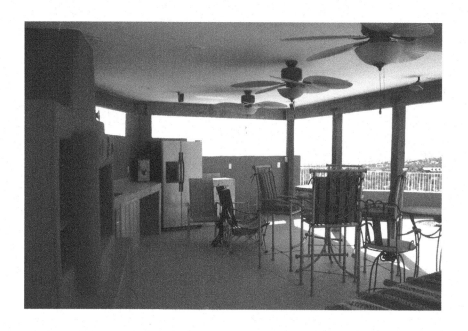

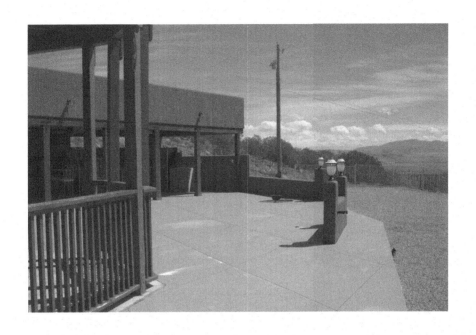

You can reach Sam's

ALL FAITH SELF-HELP CENTER

by logging onto
www.sammeranto.com

or by telephone at
602-957-4669 or 1-800-580-5080

Physical Address
4440 East Indian School Road
Phoenix, AZ 85018

September 22, 2011

I've known Sam Meranto for about twenty years, and I've watched him work with hundreds of people. He has a natural gift. It's not something you learn in medical school. He's been helping people all over the country since the 1950s. It's amazing to me where he gets the stamina to continue helping people. He has created about 1,600 stereo audio recordings on every subject you can imagine. He has taught his staff to read the 225-question evaluation and find in his library the sessions that pinpoint the areas people need help in. This method is far superior to anything I have witnessed before. They will continue helping people until the end of time.

Dr. Lewis Heller, MD

April 22, 2012 the Arizona Republic (tenth largest newspaper in the US) wrote a three page story on Sam Meranto. You can look it up on azcentral.com on the internet. They have a video of Sam in his office. It is titled "An 80 year old can make love everyday if he wants to". Look it up. They did a story about him being in business for 35 years in the same office. They also checked the better business bureau and found only one complaint in 35 years. This is a record that is amazing and unbelievable, considering almost 20,000 people have taken Sam's course and only one complaint. The article went on to say that Sam was the father of 6 kids and divorced which happened forty years ago. It reported that Sam spent 35 years trying to get into people's minds. That's 100 percent true. By doing so he changed people's lives. Some clients lost over 100 pounds and even came back after 30 years to tell of their continued success. People got over alcoholism after rehabs failed. Others have been in pain clinics, sleep clinics and spent thousands and thousands of dollars to no avail. The doctors tried many different modalities and everything failed, until Sam Meranto got them positive help. The reporter was right Sam did get into their minds and made the changes they needed.

The reporter made fun of Sam's video productions, which are not Hollywood productions phonied up with actors. Sam's videos are real people with real problems and true stories. They had to agree to be on TV and sign a release. Some people are private and choose not to tell their success story. Sam is grateful to all the people that agreed to share their experiences, because they give encouragement to people like them.

Like myself, Sam's sessions helped me to lose 50 pounds and get over depression that started in my childhood. He was also able to help my daughter who was born with a lack of oxygen to her brain resulting in developmental disabilities. Sam did a regression where he regressed her back into the womb and the results are amazing. She is in school and even recently got married.

Last week I saw a play that Jesse Kove starred in, a son of a famous movie star, Martin Kove (Karate Kid & Cagney and Lacy). Marty brought Jesse in to see Sam ten years ago for ADD. He wouldn't get up in the morning and was getting in trouble frequently. Even though he was not quite four feet tall he was somewhat of a bully. Six months went by, after coming in to see Sam, and Jesse was brought back to tell of his success. Sam gave him a microphone and videotaped him. In his own words Jesse was explaining to Sam how his grades improved, he was getting up in the mornings, being nicer to other kids, and told Sam that he wanted to be a Director. Sam said, "No you are going to be a movie star like your father".

Jesse came to Sam's office recently. He now stands 6'4" and has been in 6 movies and starred in some New York stage plays. Look for his name, Jesse Kove, Sam predicts he is going to be a major movie star.

What about your kids or grandkids? Sam has made recordings to help them in school, to stop bullying, stay away from gangs, alcohol and drugs. You can call the toll free number, 800-580-5080 to find out how to get these sessions. You can also download a session from the website sammeranto.com. We can even call you after you have filled out the Lifestyle Analysis. Mail it in, because you don't want your business on the internet. Everything is confidential (like going to a priest or minister). Sam's office is a spiritual counseling center. Here is your chance to get things off your chest and get the help you need.

THE ARIZONA REPUBLIC STORY

It is highly likely that if you live in the Phoenix area, you have seen Sam Meranto on television, and it is highly likely that you didn't plan to. For more than 30 years, Meranto, calls himself the king of mind power.

Perhaps it's 2 a.m. and you can't sleep. Perhaps it's 2 p.m. and you're flipping through daytime television before the kids get home from school. Sam Meranto is standing there in front of a blue background, clad in a suit jacket with no tie, and he would like to help you with whatever is weighing on your mind.

"If you're overweight, if you're drinking, if you got a sexual problem, you're not making enough money ... you can correct it by using what God gave you, and that's your mind," Meranto tells the camera in a thick East Coast accent.

The commercial cuts to a series of low-production-value, quick-edit testimonials. Here's Christine, who lost 80 pounds, Mary Lou, who stopped smoking, Mike quit drinking, and here's Pete, who was able to throw away his pain medication. The clips are also a trip through a hair and fashion time machine. Meranto recycles some testimonials for decades, mixing them with others that could have been shot last Tuesday.

He works to help people, hoping that either your insomnia or your daytime boredom, coupled with your weight or your paycheck or your lack of motivation, find the help they deserve.

"Folks, come in for a free session and a free consultation," he says, looking into the camera. "I've been in the same location for 35 years. That must say something."

It does say something that the now 80-year-old Meranto has been here that long; convincing people they can change even lifelong problems by donning headphones and listening repeatedly to his prerecorded therapy sessions. What it says — about Meranto... is worth exploring.

Since 1977, Meranto has been able to convince plenty of Arizonans, mainly through TV commercials, that he can "put a new head on them" through a mixture of biblical quotations, common-sense advice and hypnotic sound effects. His best proof that his methods work is the video recordings of those patients who agree to be in his commercials, talking about their successes.

"I have a natural gift. I don't know what it is," he said during an interview in his office, situated on Indian School Road...

A prospective client coming to Meranto's office is greeted by a large television playing a continuous loop of his commercials and infomercials. On the walls are about 60 photographs of Meranto shaking hands with various celebrities — Donny and Marie Osmond, Chuck Connors, Charlton Heston, Ernest Borgnine — showing that he has hobnobbed with the greats... he has helped quite a few, like Tom Jones, Donald O'Conner, Angie Dickenson, and Marie Osmond for loss of a loved one, just to name a few.

Clients are led to the "therapy room," a darkened space with leather recliners, and given headphones to listen to an introductory session in which Meranto explains how his recordings work. "Folks, this program is powerful," he says. "I want you to get help and Satan doesn't want you to get help.

The prospective clients are asked to fill out a 225-question survey — questions about depression, weight, relationship with mother, age difference between parents, among other things — and they watch a video in which Meranto says he can "reprogram" their brains to erase their trauma.

"I can empty mental institutions and have the doctors looking for jobs," he says on the video. He also mentions the cost and encourages them to sign up. When they sign up, a person has access to the library of more than 1,600 sessions that Meranto has recorded over the years. The CDs line the wall of his production facility, sorted by problem and arranged on spindles nailed to a pegboard wall.

"People come out, they say, 'Where do I sign?'" Meranto said.

THE PROGRAM

Meranto records his sessions in one take without a script, not stopping even for technical glitches... "I flub a word, I twist a grammar, but you know it's like I'm sitting with you," he said.

He believes that his method is the reverse of psychotherapy, where patients are the ones who talk out their problems. Instead, Meranto's clients don headphones, relax, maybe even fall asleep, and Meranto does all the talking.

"I tell people, 'Shut your mouth up and put a zipper on it,'" he said.

While they're in that relaxed state, Meranto says, he implants his "suggestions," which, to the conscious mind, sound more like practical advice.

"I talk to them like a Dutch uncle," he said.

He takes a client back to childhood, prodding memories about how their parents spoke to them about food.

"Success breeds success," Meranto says. "Smell the success in your childhood. If you listen to this tape a number of times, you won't remember the poverty you went through."

" Meranto's success rate is unclear, but official complaints are few for someone who has been in business for 35 years. Better Business Bureau online records show only one complaint lodged against the company in those years.

"Let me put it this way," Meranto said. "When it doesn't work, they let you know, and I get very few people that do that."

THE EARLY YEARS

It's no surprise that Meranto's first jobs were in sales.

Growing up in Niagara Falls, N.Y., during the Great Depression, he went door-to-door with his grandmother's homemade cheese. He later toted his own shoeshine box. By age 6, he said, his father took him to his work at a used-car lot.

"I'd sit on the fender while my father was showing the cars," Meranto said.

His father died when Meranto was 7. When Meranto's mother remarried, the man moved the family to Worcester, Mass. It was there that, as a teenager during a troop meeting of the Sea Scouts, Meranto was first exposed to hypnotism. A fellow Scout called him to the front to put him under, using the traditional swaying watch. Meranto didn't fall under the spell, but he became intrigued with the possibilities.

That was about all he studied. His asthma caused him to miss a lot of school, Meranto said, and teachers would throw him out of class for talking. He dropped out after his sophomore year in high school and began working, selling Fuller Brushes door-to-door, and then, at 18, Electrolux vacuum cleaners.

To inspire himself, Meranto made a recording. "I just told myself, 'You're going to make five sales a day.'" And he became one of Electrolux's top salesmen, he said.

In June 1953, a tornado swept through a Worcester neighborhood where he was selling vacuums. Just before the storm hit, Meranto had been ready to quit for the day, but something told him to try to make one more sale. Had he not pressed on, he believes he would have been caught up in the tornado that killed 94 people.

"My life was spared to do the work I'm doing now," he said. Although he didn't grow up with much religion, he says the terrifying event made him a believer in Jesus Christ.

Meranto married at 18 and had six kids, but the couple divorced in 1971. In the settlement, he had to sell a school he had started in the late 1960s for heavy-equipment drivers, and, with the cash, decided to come to Arizona. He was 40 at the time.

"I always wanted to go to Arizona," he said, citing his love for Western movies. "Gene Autry, Roy Rogers ... I'm a cowboy."

THE SUCCESS STORIES

Never camera-shy, Meranto was among the first to use long-form television advertising. Surrounded by a roomful of successful clients at his first taping, he spoke for three hours with no script. It was winnowed down to an hour, which aired on Channel 45 in 1987.

He keeps a thick, three-ring binder filled with clippings and photographs of past patients, and will turn to any page and tell the story of the people pictured. Meranto flipped the binder to a clipping of professional golfer Jim Ahern, for instance, who hadn't had much success on the PGA Tour and was about to try the Senior Tour. Meranto told Ahern that he would be a winning golfer and, as Meranto tells it, six months later Ahern won his first tournament, netting $1.3million.

Reached by phone, Ahern, 63, backed up Meranto's story. He said he had heard about Meranto through his infomercials and commercials, and that the sessions helped him get his first win.

On the wall of his lobby, Meranto has a photo of Matt Williams, the former Arizona Diamondbacks third baseman, sitting in a therapy chair in the fall of 2002. Meranto said Williams came to him to give up chewing tobacco and that Meranto helped him not only to kick that habit, but also to improve his hitting.

Meranto flipped to another page and showed a September 1996 clipping from Life magazine. The cover story headlined "The Healing Revolution," discussed medical doctors' increasing use of alternative treatments. One of the doctors quoted was Sam Benjamin, an author and radio-show host, who, Meranto pointed out, used to work for him at the center.

From his Scottsdale office, Benjamin said that, at the time, Meranto was looking for physicians who would give quick physicals to incoming clients. Benjamin, fresh out of medical school, was young and needed the money. He had been interested in alternative healing techniques and was intrigued at seeing people walk out of Meranto's office with changed lives.

"In some context, he's giving them time and words and caring," said Benjamin, whose own practice includes meditation and natural herbs. "We oftentimes neglect ... how important it is to have a positive approach to whatever emotional or physical problem there might be," he said.

Benjamin appeared in one of Meranto's commercials with an endorsement, saying Meranto's methods "do no harm." "That's what he's telling people," Benjamin said. "What's so terrible?"

To Meranto, though, his approach is more revolutionary than that. He believes it constitutes a unique way of reprogramming the human mind, reversing bad habits and erasing old traumas, he said. That's why he doesn't understand why he's never really gotten the recognition that befits such an innovator.

"You look at Christopher Columbus, they said he was a wacko," Meranto said. Similarly, he said, perhaps his theories about the mind might be too radical to be appreciated in his own time.

"I'm saying the mind is simple, easy to understand," Meranto said. "They make it complicated."

THE WIND DOWN

Meranto often points to himself as his own best client, touting himself as a model for living. At 80, he remains in good shape, lifts weights, is mentally sharp and claims he is able to make love every day, a boast that causes his wife, Cynthia, 51, if she is in the room, to blush slightly.

When he eventually retires, Meranto sees himself relaxing, hitting the open road in the recreational vehicle currently parked in his backyard. He wants to visit relatives back in Massachusetts before it's too late. He just lost a sister. And his brother, who weighed 400 pounds and resisted Meranto's efforts to diet, passed away at age 67.

"When I'm retired," he said, "there'll be nobody left to go visit."

He does find himself thinking about retiring from time to time, but can't quite bring himself to do it. His business is not yet self-sustaining without his presence. He fears that if he stopped working, his legacy would suddenly disappear, like a hypnotic suggestion at the snap of a finger.

"For a guy who does the good work that I do, I should have millions of dollars," he said. Meranto was sitting at his editing bay, having hit the pause on a tape of old testimonials. "I get people out of wheelchairs. No one throws a big party for me."

"If I could get people under my spell, I wouldn't be working at 80," he said, his voice rising over the relaxing music. "I'd have a ton of money. I don't," he said. There was a slight pause. "Because I love my work."

Meranto has slowly prepared to step away. There's a for-sale sign on one of his properties, a building he had once hoped to turn into a Hispanic outreach center. He's also recently sold the All-Faith building and his thousands of recorded sessions to his non-profit charity, each a $1 million transaction, marking his biggest sales.

He watches for someone who could take over his business, maybe even set up franchises across the country. But in truth, he figures that, like Elvis Presley, the Meranto name might be more well-known after his death, which would give sales of his CD sessions a postmortem bump.

"And they're going to work better," he said of the sessions, "because I'm going to be up there with God, saying to him, 'Hey, make that work better.'"